Hematology Outlines
Atlas and Glossary
of Hematology

Hooman H. Rashidi, MD
Author and Editor

John C. Nguyen, MD
Author and Illustrator

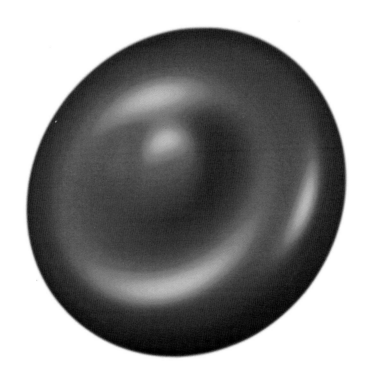

R & N
Academic
Press

Hematology Outlines: Atlas and Glossary of Hematology

First Edition Copyright © 2017 by R&N Academic Press

Disclaimer: Care has been taken to confirm the accuracy of the information presented and to describe generally accepted practices. However, the authors, editors, and publisher are not responsible for errors or omissions or for any consequences from application of the information in this book and make no warranty, expressed or implied, with respect to the currency, completeness, or accuracy of the contents of the publication. If the information is to be used for clinical practice, verification of the material with reference textbooks, accepted clinical guidelines, and/or journals is necessary. Application of this information in a particular situation remains the professional responsibility of the practitioner.

ISBN-10: 0-692-95939-4
ISBN-13: 978-0-692-95939-8
R&N Academic Press
United States of America

TABLE OF CONTENTS

ABOUT US

Hooman H. Rashidi, MD
U.C. Davis School of Medicine

I dedicate this book to my best friend and wife Kristen. Without your support none of this would have been possible.

John C. Nguyen, MD
Singlera Genomics, Medical Director

To my wonderful wife Natalie and my beautiful daughter Alanna, thank you both for your endless support and for always being guiding lights in my life and our endeavours.

The Hematology atlas and glossary in which this print version is based on was first introduced and integrated into the Hematology course at UC San Diego School of Medicine. Thereafter it became an integral part of the Hematology/Hematopathology course at UC Davis School of Medicine. It has also been integrated into the hematology course curriculum at various medical schools and Clinical Laboratory Scientist (CLS) training programs. The online and App versions (accessible at http://www.hematologyoutlines.com) have received the highest reviews and have been used by students, residents, fellows and practitioners in the United States and abroad with over 200,000 users since its inception. It has also been an American Society of Clinical Pathology (ASCP) recommended suggested reading reference for Hematology certification for Specialists in Hematology and Technologists in Hematology since 2013. This print version is a result of multiple student requests and incorporates the best of our online version with certain added features.

We hope you find it useful in your educational endeavors.

- Hooman H. Rashidi MD & John C. Nguyen MD

✳ RECOGNITIONS ✳

- The online website and the iPhone and Android Apps (accessible at http://www.hematologyoutlines.com) have been consistently in the top of the online Hematology atlases and apps.
- It is also an ASCP recommended resource for Hematology certification.
- The Atlas and Glossary are now officially a part of the Hematology course in multiple medical schools and clinical laboratory scientist (CLS) training programs.

CONTRIBUTORS

This print version is based on the online and App versions (accessible at http://www.hematologyoutlines.com). Contributors to the Hematology Outlines Atlas and Glossary (online and App versions) include:

Hooman H. Rashidi, MD
University of California, Davis School of Medicine

John C. Nguyen, MD
Singlera Genomics, Inc., Medical Director

Erin Reid, MD
University of California, San Diego School of Medicine

David Li, MD
University of Utah School of Medicine

Huan-You Wang, MD, PhD
University of California, San Diego School of Medicine

Michael J. Borowitz, MD, PhD
Johns Hopkins School of Medicine

Demitrios Braddock MD, PhD
Yale University, School of Medicine

Sheeja Pullarkat, MD
University of California Los Angeles, School of Medicine

Antonio Galvao Neto, MD
NYU School of Medicine

Robert Sharpe, MD
Scripps Clinic, La Jolla, CA

Anna K. Wong, MD
DPMG, Sacramento, CA

John Blaustein, MD
Cottage Hospital, Santa Barbara, CA

Arash Mohtashamian, MD
Naval Hospital, San Diego CA

Brett M. Mahon, MD
Rush University, School of Medicine

Jeff Truell, MD
Swedish Medical Center, Colorado

Nathan Yee, MD
University of Washington, School of Medicine

Don Xu, MD, PhD
University of California, San Diego School of Medicine

James C. Valentine MD
Naval Hospital, San Diego CA

Sepi Mahooti, MD
University of California, San Diego School of Medicine

Elham Vali-Betts, MD
University of California, Davis School of Medicine

Copy Editor: Hirbod Rashidi, JD
University of California, Riverside (Extension)
University of California, Los Angeles (Extension)

TUTORIAL

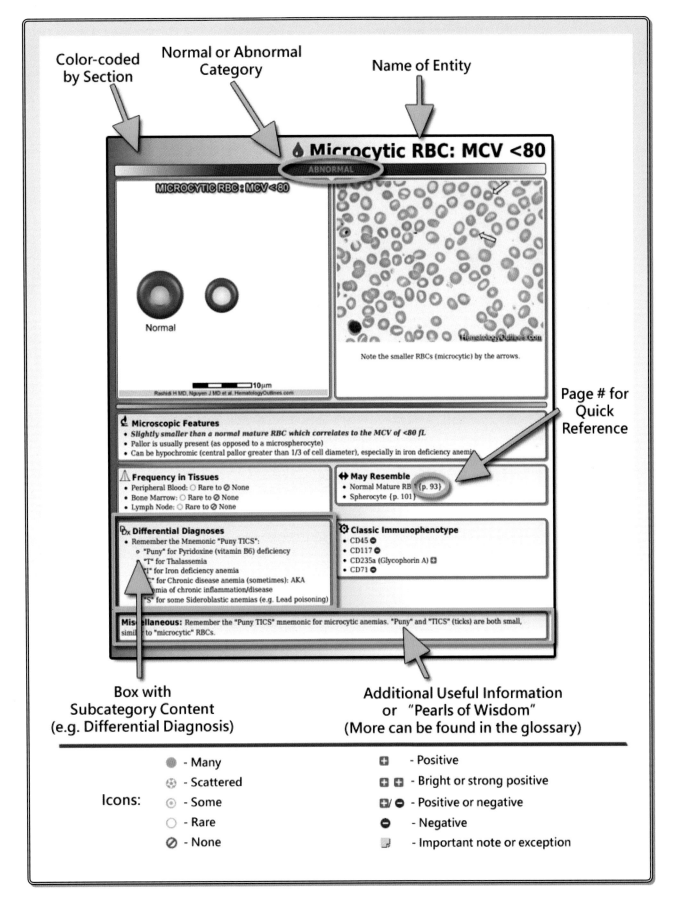

Color-coded by Section

Normal or Abnormal Category

Name of Entity

🜆 **Microcytic RBC: MCV <80**

ABNORMAL

MICROCYTIC RBC: MCV <80

Normal

⊢10µm

Rashidi H MD, Nguyen J MD et al. HematologyOutlines.com

Note the smaller RBCs (microcytic) by the arrows.

Page # for Quick Reference

🔬 **Microscopic Features**
- *Slightly smaller than a normal mature RBC which correlates to the MCV of <80 fL*
- Pallor is usually present (as opposed to a microspherocyte)
- Can be hypochromic (central pallor greater than 1/3 of cell diameter), especially in iron deficiency anemia

⚠ **Frequency in Tissues**
- Peripheral Blood: ○ Rare to ⊘ None
- Bone Marrow: ○ Rare to ⊘ None
- Lymph Node: ○ Rare to ⊘ None

↔ **May Resemble**
- Normal Mature RBC {p. 93}
- Spherocyte {p. 101}

℞ₓ **Differential Diagnoses**
- Remember the Mnemonic "Puny TICS":
  - "Puny" for Pyridoxine (vitamin B6) deficiency
  - "T" for Thalassemia
  - "I" for Iron deficiency anemia
  - "C" for Chronic disease anemia (sometimes): AKA anemia of chronic inflammation/disease
  - "S" for some Sideroblastic anemias (e.g. Lead poisoning)

⚙ **Classic Immunophenotype**
- CD45 ⊖
- CD117 ⊖
- CD235a (Glycophorin A) ⊞
- CD71 ⊖

Miscellaneous: Remember the "Puny TICS" mnemonic for microcytic anemias. "Puny" and "TICS" (ticks) are both small, similar to "microcytic" RBCs.

Box with Subcategory Content (e.g. Differential Diagnosis)

Additional Useful Information or "Pearls of Wisdom" (More can be found in the glossary)

Icons:

● - Many	⊞ - Positive
⊛ - Scattered	⊞ ⊞ - Bright or strong positive
◉ - Some	⊞/⊖ - Positive or negative
○ - Rare	⊖ - Negative
⊘ - None	🗒 - Important note or exception

ATLAS OVERVIEW MINDMAP

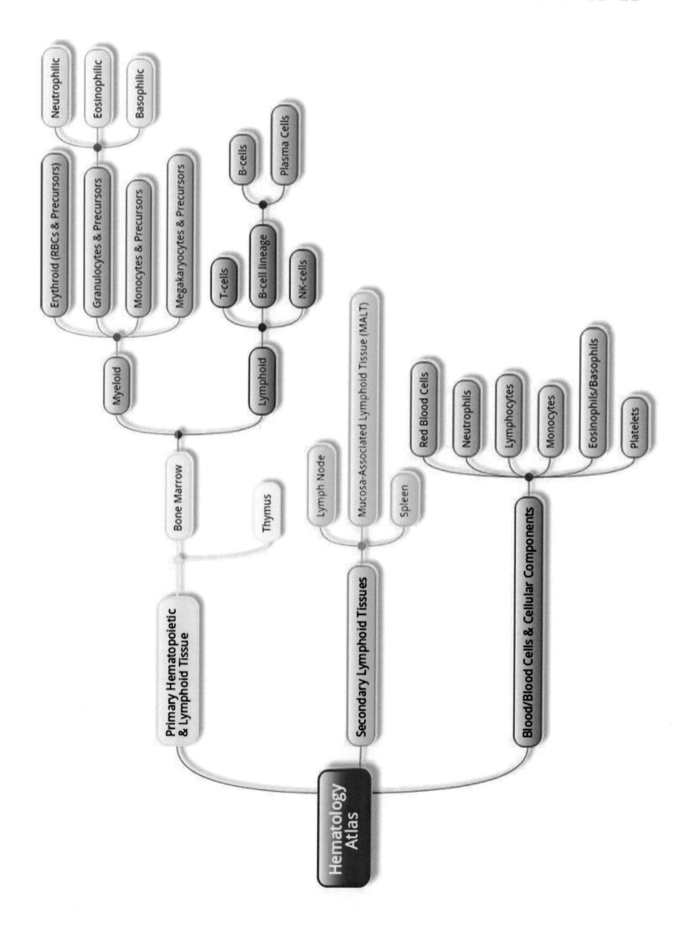

Bone Marrow: Myeloid Overview Mindmap

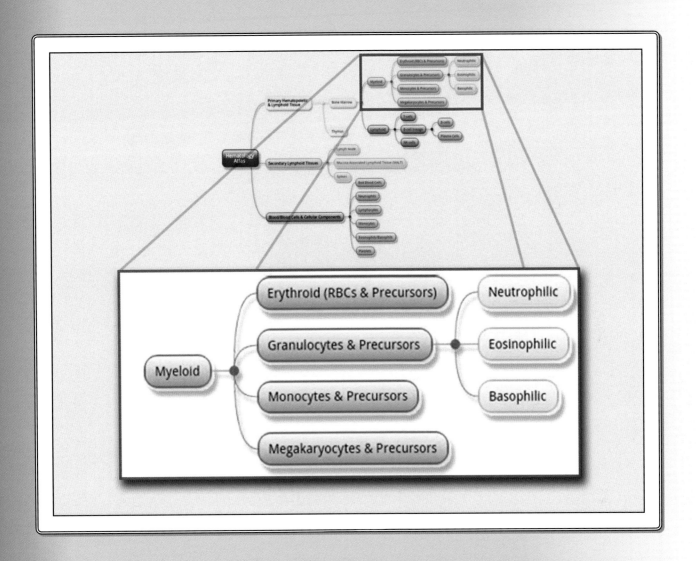

Erythrocyte (RBC) Maturation Diagram

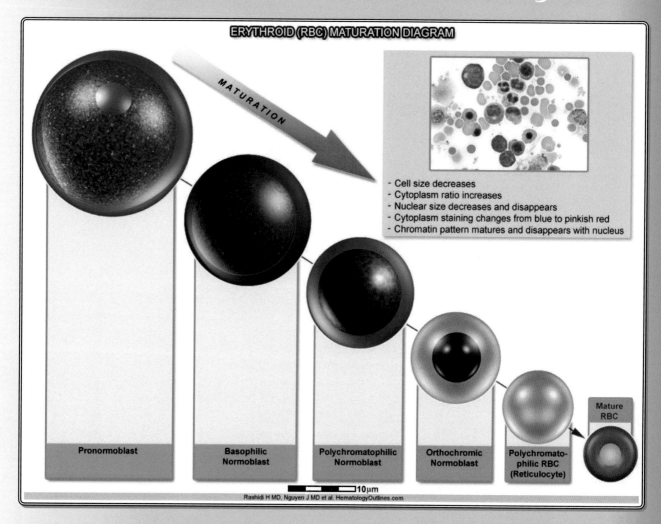

ERYTHROID (RBC) MATURATION DIAGRAM

MATURATION

- Cell size decreases
- Cytoplasm ratio increases
- Nuclear size decreases and disappears
- Cytoplasm staining changes from blue to pinkish red
- Chromatin pattern matures and disappears with nucleus

Mature RBC

Pronormoblast | Basophilic Normoblast | Polychromatophilic Normoblast | Orthochromic Normoblast | Polychromato-philic RBC (Reticulocyte)

10µm

Rashidi H MD, Nguyen J MD et al. HematologyOutlines.com

The goal of the erythroid maturation process is to give rise to the mature red blood cell (RBC). Ultimately this is accomplished by losing its nucleus and increasing its hemoglobin content to maximize the RBC's oxygen carrying capacity. Understanding this normal maturation process is essential in understanding RBC disorders.

🩸 **Pronormoblast**

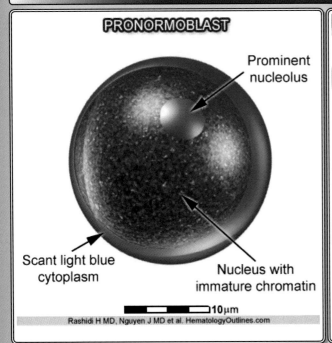

PRONORMOBLAST

Prominent nucleolus

Scant light blue cytoplasm

Nucleus with immature chromatin

⊨▬▬▬▬⊐10µm

Rashidi H MD, Nguyen J MD et al. HematologyOutlines.com

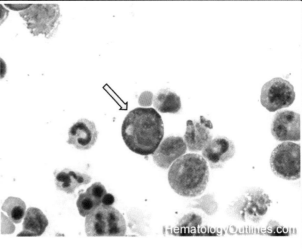

Bone marrow aspirate
Note the larger cell size, prominent nucleoli, and rim of blue cytoplasm.

🔬 Microscopic Features
- 3-4X larger than a mature RBC
- High nuclear-to-cytoplasmic (N/C) ratio
- Round nucleus with immature chromatin (not clumped)
- *Prominent nucleoli*
- Cytoplasm is scant and light blue in color

⚠️ Frequency in Tissues
- Peripheral Blood: ⊘ None
- Bone Marrow: ○ Rare
- Lymph Node: ⊘ None

↔ May Resemble
- Myeloblast {p. 21}
- Basophilic Normoblast {p. 10}
- Monoblast {p. 38}

℞x Differential Diagnoses
- ⬆ Increased in:
  - Erythroid leukemia (AML M6)
  - Polycythemia vera
  - Reactive erythroid hyperplasia

⚙ Classic Immunophenotype
- CD36 ➕ ➕
- CD117 ➕
- CD235a (Glycophorin A) ➖ to **dim** ➕
- CD71 ➕ / ➖
- E-cadherin ➕
- Hemoglobin ➖
- Aldehyde dehydrogenase ➕
- Carbonic anhydrase I ➕

Miscellaneous: In normal bone marrow, they comprise 1-2% of the total nucleated cells which is approximately 2-3% of the nucleated red blood cell precursors.

📝**Note**: As erythroid precursors mature, the color of their cytoplasm changes from blue to gray to red-orange (this is due to the increase in the number of hemoglobin molecules within the red blood cells as they mature). Additionally, the nucleus of the red blood cell becomes more dense as it matures and it eventually excretes from the cell, forming the mature red blood cell.

🔴 Basophilic Normoblast

BASOPHILIC NORMOBLAST

Round nucleus with immature chromatin

High N:C

Deep blue cytoplasm

10µm

Rashidi H MD, Nguyen J MD et al. HematologyOutlines.com

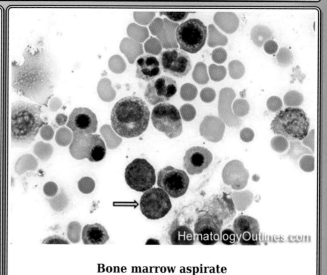

Bone marrow aspirate
The arrow depicts a basophilic normoblast in a background of erythroid and myeloid precursors in various stages of maturation.

🔬 Microscopic Features
- 2-3X larger than a mature RBC
- High nuclear-to-cytoplasmic (N/C) ratio
- Round Nucleus with immature chromatin (not clumped)
- *Nucleoli are NOT prominent*
- Cytoplasm is deep blue in color and with perinuclear clearing

⚠ Frequency in Tissues
- Peripheral Blood: ⊘ None
- Bone Marrow: ✹ Scattered
- Lymph Node: ⊘ None

↔ May Resemble
- Pronormoblast {p. 9}
- Polychromatophilic Normoblast {p. 11}
- Orthochromic Normoblast {p. 12}
- Plasma Cell Precursor (Plasmablast) {p. 69}
- Immature B-cell (hematogone) {p. 62}

Dx Differential Diagnoses
- ↑ Increased in:
  - Polycythemia vera
  - Post-erythropoietin therapy
  - Reactive erythroid hyperplasia

⚙ Classic Immunophenotype
- CD36 ➕ ➕
- CD45 **dim** ➕ to ➖
- CD34 ➖ and Hemoglobin ➖
- CD117 ➕ and CD71 ➕
- CD235a (Glycophorin A) **very dim** ➕
- E-cadherin ➕

Miscellaneous: In normal marrow they comprise 2-3% of the total nucleated cells which is approximately 5-8% of the nucleated red blood cells precursors.

📝**Note**: As erythroid precursors mature, the color of their cytoplasm changes from blue to gray to red-orange (this is due to the increase in the number of hemoglobin molecules within the red cells as they mature). Additionally, the nucleus of the red blood cell will become more dense as it matures, eventually excreting from the cell forming the mature RBC.

⬥ Polychromatophilic Normoblast

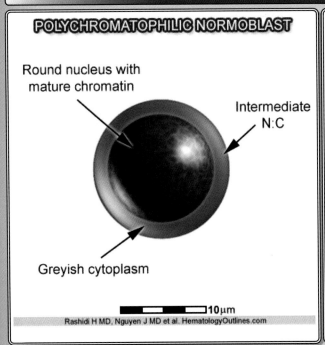

POLYCHROMATOPHILIC NORMOBLAST

Round nucleus with mature chromatin

Intermediate N:C

Greyish cytoplasm

10μm

Rashidi H MD, Nguyen J MD et al. HematologyOutlines.com

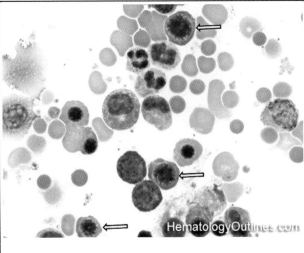

Bone marrow aspirate
The yellow arrows point to the polychromatophilic normoblasts in a background of erythroid and myeloid precursors in various stages of maturation.

⚗ Microscopic Features
- 2X larger than a mature RBC
- Intermediate nuclear-to-cytoplasmic (N:C) ratio
- Round nucleus with mature chromatin (clumped)
- *Nucleoli are absent*
- Cytoplasm is grayish in color

⚠ Frequency in Tissues
- Peripheral Blood: ⊘ None
- Bone Marrow: ● Many
- Lymph Node: ⊘ None

↔ May Resemble
- Orthochromic Normoblast {p. 12}
- Plasma Cell (mature) {p. 67}
- Basophilic Normoblast {p. 10}
- Lymphocyte (mature) {p. 64}

℞ Differential Diagnoses
- ↑ Increased in:
  - Reactive erythroid hyperplasia
  - Post-erythropoietin therapy
  - Polycythemia vera

⚙ Classic Immunophenotype
- CD36 ⊞ ⊞
- CD45 ⊖
- CD117 ⊖
- CD235a (Glycophorin A) ⊞
- CD71 ⊞
- Hemoglobin ⊞

Miscellaneous: Polychromatophilic normoblasts are normally confined to the bone marrow where they comprise many of the nucleated red blood cell precursors.

♪ Note: As erythroid precursors mature, the color of their cytoplasm changes from blue to gray to red-orange (this is due to the increase in number of hemoglobin molecules within the red blood cells as they mature). Additionally, the nucleus of the red blood cell will become more dense as it matures, eventually excreting from the cell forming the mature red blood cell.

⬤ Orthochromatophilic Normoblast

NORMAL

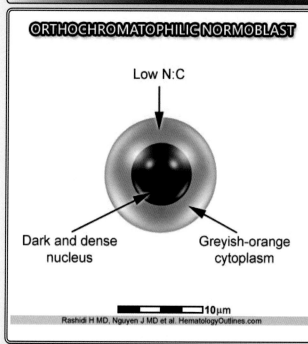

ORTHOCHROMATOPHILIC NORMOBLAST

Low N:C

Dark and dense nucleus

Greyish-orange cytoplasm

10µm

Rashidi H MD, Nguyen J MD et al. HematologyOutlines.com

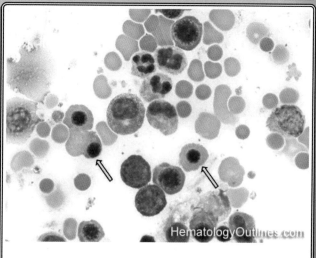

HematologyOutlines.com

Bone marrow aspirate

The yellow arrows point to the orthochromatophilic normoblasts in a background of erythroid and myeloid precursors in various stages of maturation.

🔬 Microscopic Features
- 1.5 - 2X larger than a mature RBC
- Low nuclear-to-cytoplasmic (N:C) ratio
- *Round nucleus (sometimes eccentric) with pyknotic chromatin (dark and dense)*
- Nucleoli are NOT seen
- Cytoplasm is grayish-orange in color

⚠ Frequency in Tissues
- Peripheral Blood: ⊘ None
- Bone Marrow: ⬤ Many
- Lymph Node: ⊘ None

↔ May Resemble
- Lymphocyte (mature) {p. 64}
- Polychromatophilic Normoblast {p. 11}
- Plasma Cell {p. 67}

ᴅx Differential Diagnoses
- ⬆ Increased in:
  - Reactive erythroid hyperplasia
  - Post-erythropoietin therapy
  - Polycythemia vera

⚙ Classic Immunophenotype
- CD36 ➕
- CD45 ➖
- CD117 ➖
- Hemoglobin ➕
- CD235a (Glycophorin A) ➕ ➕
- CD71 ➕ / ➖

Miscellaneous: Orthochromatophilic normoblasts are normally confined to the bone marrow where they comprise many of the nucleated red blood cell precursors.

Note: As erythroid precursors mature, the color of their cytoplasm changes from blue to gray to red-orange (this is due to the increase in number of hemoglobin molecules within the red blood cells as they mature). Additionally, the nucleus of the red blood cell will become more dense as it matures, eventually excreting from the cell forming the mature red blood cell.

◖ Polychromatophilic RBC

POLYCHROMATOPHILIC RED BLOOD CELL (RETICULOCYTE WITH SPECIAL STAIN)

Called a reticulocyte when precipitated RNA can be highlighted with supravital stain

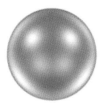

Lacks a nucleus

▬▬▬□▬□**10μm**

Rashidi H MD, Nguyen J MD et al. HematologyOutlines.com

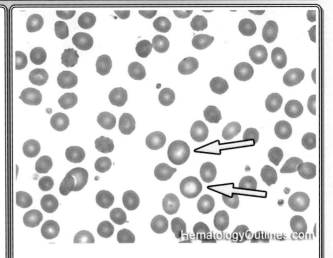

Note the slightly larger RBCs at the yellow arrows. These polychromatophilic RBCs are slightly less mature and have a greyish color (due to RNA).

🔬 Microscopic Features
- *Slightly larger than normal mature RBCs*
- Lacks a nucleus
- Cytoplasm is greyish-orange in color (since it is less mature than a normal mature RBC)

⚠ Frequency in Tissues
- Peripheral Blood: 1-2%
- Bone Marrow: ✪ Scattered
- Lymph Node: ○ Rare to ⊘ None

↔ May Resemble
- With normal stain (not supravital) may resemble:
  - Mature RBC {p. 91}
  - Macrocytic RBC {p. 95}
  - Giant Platelet {p. 155} (especially if hypogranular)
- Reticulocyte (with supravital stain) may resemble:
  - Heinz Bodies {p. 110}
  - RBC with stain artifact

℞ Differential Diagnoses
- ⬆ Increased in:
  - Response to some anemias (e.g. hemolytic anemia or blood loss)
  - Reactive erythroid hyperplasia
  - Post erythropoietin (EPO) therapy
  - Polycythemia vera
  - May be increased in newborns

⚙ Classic Immunophenotype
- Hemoglobin ⊞
- CD45 ⊖
- CD117 ⊖
- CD235a (Glycophorin A) ⊞
- CD71 ⊖

Miscellaneous: A polychromatophilic red blood cell is called a reticulocyte when a supravital stain highlights the precipitated RNA.

🩸 Normal Mature Red Blood Cell

NORMAL MATURE RED BLOOD CELL

Central pallor is
1/3 diameter

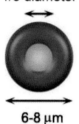

6-8 μm

10μm

Rashidi, MD & Nguyen, MD et al. HematologyOutlines.com

central pallor is
~1/3 diameter

HematologyOutlines.com

Peripheral blood smear
Laying flat, the red blood cell can be equally divided
into thirds by the size of the central pallor.

🔬 Microscopic Features
- Size 6-8 μm, slightly smaller than a mature lymphocyte
- *Lacks a nucleus*
- Cytoplasm is pink-orange in color with a central pallor
- Central pallor is 1/3 the diameter

⚠ Frequency in Tissues
- Peripheral blood: 🔴 Many
- Bone marrow: 🔴 Many
- Lymphoid tissue: ◉ Some

↔ May Resemble
- Polychromatophilic RBC {p. 13}
- Macrocytic RBC {p. 95}
- Microcytic RBC {p. 94}
- Giant Platelet {p. 155}

Dx Differential Diagnoses
- ↑ Increased in:
  - Reactive erythroid hyperplasia
  - Post-erythropoietin therapy
  - Polycythemia vera

⚙ Classic Immunophenotype
- Hemoglobin ➕
- CD45 ➖
- CD117 ➖
- CD235a (Glycophorin A) ➕
- CD71 ➖

Miscellaneous: Normal mature RBCs are normocytic (MCV 80-100 μm) and normochromic (~1/3 central pallor). Its main function is to carry oxygen via its hemoglobin molecules.

Note: As erythroid precursors mature, the color of their cytoplasm changes from blue to gray to red-orange (this is due to the increase in the number of hemoglobin molecules within the red blood cells as they mature). Additionally, the nucleus of the red blood cell will become more dense as it matures, eventually excreting from the cell forming the mature red blood cell.

⬥ Ring Sideroblast

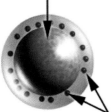

RINGED SIDEROBLAST

Round nucleus with no nucleous

Iron Stain:

Iron granules
(5 or more encircling
> 1/3 of the nucleus

10µm

Rashidi H MD, Nguyen J MD et al. HematologyOutlines.com

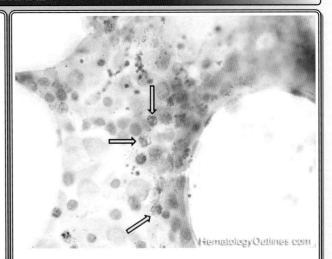

Iron stain of bone marrow aspirate
The yellow arrows point to the ring sideroblasts.

🔬 Microscopic Features
- Size is variable depending on the stage of maturation
- Nuclear-to-cytoplasmic ratio (N:C) is variable depending on the stage of maturation
- Round nucleus
- Nucleoli are NOT visible
- *Iron deposits are visualized with an iron stain as blue granules (5 or more granules that encircle >1/3 of the nucleus)*

⚠ Frequency in Tissues
- Peripheral Blood: ⊘ None
- Bone Marrow: ⊘ None
- Lymph Node: ⊘ None

↔ May Resemble
- Sideroblast is similar on iron stain but with less than 5 granules

℞x Differential Diagnoses
- ↑ Increased in:
  - Zinc toxicity (may be secondary to induced copper deficiency)
  - MDS (e.g. Refractory Anemia with Ring Sideroblast)
  - States of iron overload such as hemochromatosis (sometimes)

⚙ Classic Immunophenotype
- CD45 ⊖
- CD117 ⊖
- CD235a (Glycophorin A) **dim** ⊞
- CD71 ⊞
- **Note**: The immunoprofile can be variable and may show aberrancies

Miscellaneous: Normally no more than 5 siderosomes (inclusions) are present per cell. Hence, a ring sideroblast is an **abnormal** finding.

◊ Dysplastic Nucleated RBC

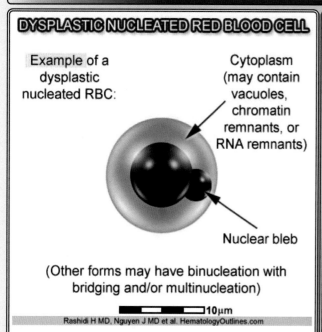

DYSPLASTIC NUCLEATED RED BLOOD CELL

Example of a dysplastic nucleated RBC:

Cytoplasm (may contain vacuoles, chromatin remnants, or RNA remnants)

Nuclear bleb

(Other forms may have binucleation with bridging and/or multinucleation)

10µm

Rashidi H MD, Nguyen J MD et al. HematologyOutlines.com

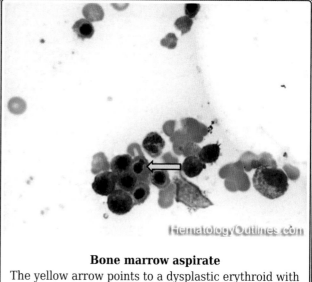

Bone marrow aspirate
The yellow arrow points to a dysplastic erythroid with nuclear blebbing.

🔬 Microscopic Features
- Size is variable depending on the stage of maturation
- Nuclear to cytoplasmic dyssynchrony may be seen
- ***Nucleus may have irregularities such as blebbing, binucleation with bridging and multinucleation***
- Cytoplasm may contain vacuoles, chromatin remnants (Howell-Jolly bodies), or RNA remnants (basophilic stippling)

⚠ Frequency in Tissues
- Peripheral Blood: ⊘ None
- Bone Marrow: ⊘ None
- Lymph Node: ⊘ None

↔ May Resemble
- Polychromatophilic Normoblast {p. 11}
- Orthochromic Normoblast {p. 12}
- Lymphocyte (mature) {p. 64}
- RBC With Howell-Jolly Body {p. 109}

Dx Differential Diagnoses
- Myelodysplastic syndrome (MDS)
- Acute myeloid leukemia
- Toxin-induced
- Chemotherapy-induced
- Congenital dyserythropoietic anemia (CDA)

⚙ Classic Immunophenotype
- CD45 ⊖
- CD117 ⊕ / ⊖
- CD235a (Glycophorin A) **dim** ⊕
- CD71 ⊕
- **Note**: The immunoprofile can be variable and may show aberrancies

Miscellaneous: Some morphologic features are indicative of stronger evidence of dysplasia than others. Nuclear blebbing, "binucleation with bridging," and multinucleation are usually considered as dysplastic features. However, the findings must always be interpreted in the correct context.

🔴 Megaloblastoid Nucleated RBC

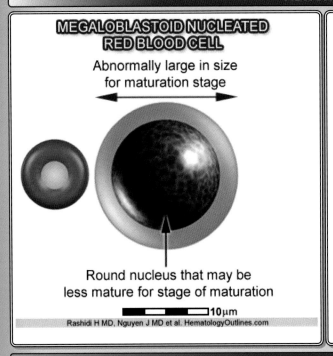

MEGALOBLASTOID NUCLEATED RED BLOOD CELL

Abnormally large in size for maturation stage

Round nucleus that may be less mature for stage of maturation

10µm

Rashidi H MD, Nguyen J MD et al. HematologyOutlines.com

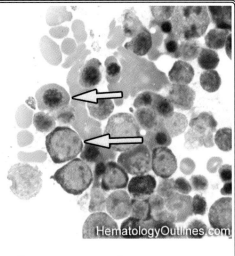

Bone marrow aspirate
The yellow arrows point to the megaloblastoid erythroids.

🔬 Microscopic Features
- *Abnormally large in size for the stage of maturation (i.e. megaloblastoid)*
- Nucleus is round and may be less mature for the stage of maturation

⚠ Frequency in Tissues
- Peripheral Blood: ⊘ None
- Bone Marrow: ⊘ None
- Lymph Node: ⊘ None

↔ May Resemble
- Pronormoblast {p. 9}
- Basophilic Normoblast {p. 10}
- Myeloblast {p. 21}
- Monocyte {p. 40}

Dx Differential Diagnoses
- B12 or folate deficiency
- Myelodysplastic syndrome (MDS)
- Acute myeloid leukemia (AML)
- Chemotherapy-induced (e.g. methotrexate)

⚙ Classic Immunophenotype
- CD45 ⊖
- CD117 ⊖ / ⊞
- CD235a (Glycophorin A) **dim** ⊞
- CD71 ⊞
- **Note**: The immunoprofile can be variable and may show aberrancies

Miscellaneous: Megaloblastoid changes are also commonly noted in non-neoplastic disorders as well (e.g. B12 or folate deficiency). Hence, interpretation of such findings should be done with extreme caution and always be interpreted in the correct context.

🩸 Nucleated RBC with Parvovirus Infection

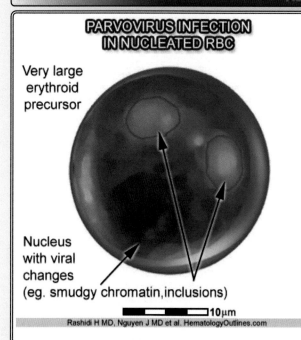

PARVOVIRUS INFECTION IN NUCLEATED RBC

Very large erythroid precursor

Nucleus with viral changes (eg. smudgy chromatin, inclusions)

▬▬▬▬10μm

Rashidi H MD, Nguyen J MD et al. HematologyOutlines.com

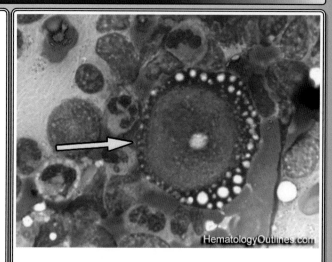

The yellow arrow points to a parvovirus-infected nucleated RBC. Note the cytoplasmic vacuoles in this case.

🔬 Microscopic Features
- *Very large erythroid precursor* with intensely blue and often vacuolated cytoplasm
- Nucleus with viral changes: Pale to moderate purple inclusion-like nucleoli or inclusions

⚠ Frequency in Tissues
- Peripheral Blood: ⊘ None
- Bone Marrow: ⊘ None
- Lymph Node: ⊘ None

↔ May Resemble
- Pronormoblast {p. 9}
- Basophilic Normoblast {p. 10}
- Myeloblast {p. 21}
- Metastatic carcinoma cells

Dx Differential Diagnoses
- Malignancy (e.g. MDS)
- CMV infection (typically involves WBCs)

⚙ Classic Immunophenotype
- Variable

Miscellaneous: A background of erythroid hypoplasia may also be present. Parvovirus B19 may be associated with aplastic anemia and pure red cell aplasia.

⬥ Erythroid Leukemia (AML M6)

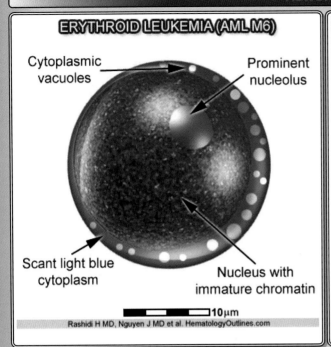

ERYTHROID LEUKEMIA (AML M6)

Cytoplasmic vacuoles

Prominent nucleolus

Scant light blue cytoplasm

Nucleus with immature chromatin

10μm

Rashidi H MD, Nguyen J MD et al. HematologyOutlines.com

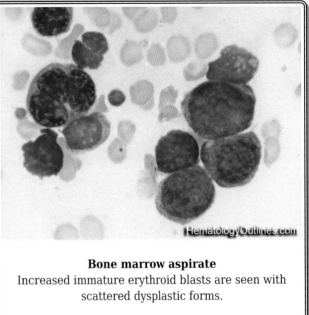

Bone marrow aspirate
Increased immature erythroid blasts are seen with scattered dysplastic forms.

🔬 Microscopic Features
- Marked increase in immature erythroid precursors
- *Background of increased erythroid precursors with dysplastic features is also common (note the multinucleated erythroid precursor on the left side of the microscopic image)*

⚠ Frequency in Tissues
- Peripheral Blood: ⊘ None
- Bone Marrow: ⊘ None
- Lymph Node: ⊘ None

↔ May Resemble
- Myeloblast {p. 21}
- Erythroid hyperplasia

ᴰx Differential Diagnoses
- Acute myeloid leukemia (other subtypes)
- Myelodysplastic syndrome (MDS)

⚙ Classic Immunophenotype
- Acute Erythroid Leukemia (Pure Erythroid-type):
  - CD45 ⊖, CD34 ⊖ and HLA-DR ⊖
  - CD117 ⊞ / ⊖ and MPO ⊖
  - CD235a (Glycophorin A) ⊞
  - Hemoglobin A ⊞
  - CD71 ⊞
  - EMA ⊞
  - PAS ⊞ / ⊖

Miscellaneous: Based on the updated WHO criteria, the diagnosis of an Acute Erythroid Leukemia (formerly known as Pure Erythroid Type) will require >80% immature erythroid precursors with ≥ 30% pronormoblasts and < 20% myeloblasts. The newly updated WHO no longer recognizes the Erythroid/Myeloid type of Erythroid Leukemia.

Granulocytic Maturation Overview Diagram

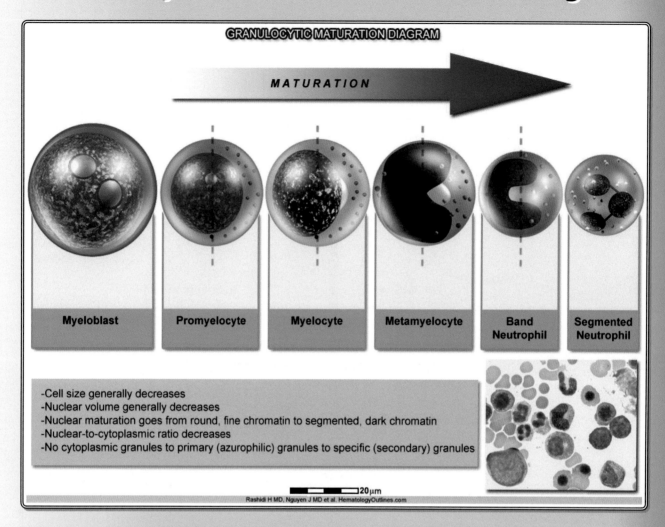

GRANULOCYTIC MATURATION DIAGRAM

MATURATION

| Myeloblast | Promyelocyte | Myelocyte | Metamyelocyte | Band Neutrophil | Segmented Neutrophil |

-Cell size generally decreases
-Nuclear volume generally decreases
-Nuclear maturation goes from round, fine chromatin to segmented, dark chromatin
-Nuclear-to-cytoplasmic ratio decreases
-No cytoplasmic granules to primary (azurophilic) granules to specific (secondary) granules

20 µm

Rashidi H MD, Nguyen J MD et al. HematologyOutlines.com

The overall trend in the series is from larger to smaller size; round, fine nucleus to dark, segmented nucleus; increasing cytoplasm; no granules to primary (azurophilic) granules to specific (secondary) granules.

NORMAL

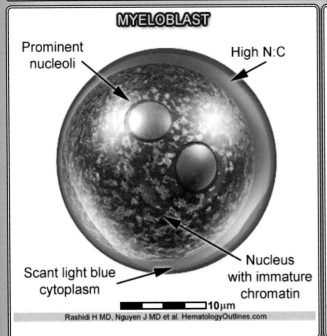

MYELOBLAST

Prominent nucleoli

High N:C

Scant light blue cytoplasm

Nucleus with immature chromatin

10μm

Rashidi H MD, Nguyen J MD et al. HematologyOutlines.com

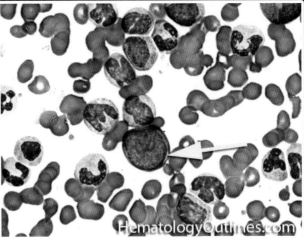

HematologyOutlines.com

Bone marrow aspirate
The yellow arrow points to a myeloblast. Notice the high N:C ratio, prominent nucleoli, and open chromatin.

🔬 Microscopic Features
- 3-4X larger than a mature RBC
- *High nuclear-to-cytoplasmic ratio (N:C)*
- Round nucleus with immature chromatin (not clumped)
- Prominent nucleoli
- Cytoplasm is scant, gray to pale blue and lacks granules

⚠ Frequency in Tissues
- Peripheral Blood: ⊘ None
- Bone Marrow: 1-3%
- Lymph Node: ⊘ None

↔ May Resemble
- Promyelocyte {p. 22}
- Pronormoblast {p. 9}
- Lymphoblast {p. 65}
- Immature B-cell (hematogone) {p. 62}
- Monoblast {p. 38}
- Reactive Lymphocyte {p. 137}

📑 Differential Diagnoses
- ⬆ Increased in:
  - Acute myeloid leukemia (AML)
  - Myelodysplastic syndromes (e.g. RAEB-I or II)
  - Myeloproliferative neoplasms (e.g. CML with increased blasts)
  - Leukemoid reactions
  - Post GCSF therapy

⚙ Classic Immunophenotype
- CD34 ➕
- CD117 ➕
- HLA-DR ➕
- CD13 ➕
- CD33 **dim** ➕
- CD15 ➖
- MPO ➖/➕

Miscellaneous: Normal bone marrow usually contains rare scattered normal myeloblasts (1-3%). A myeloblast with Auer rod(s) is by definition abnormal and usually represents an underlying AML or high grade MDS (MDS Excess Blasts 2 (MDS-EB-2) also known as Refractory Anemia with Excess Blasts 2 (RAEB-2)).

♦ Promyelocyte

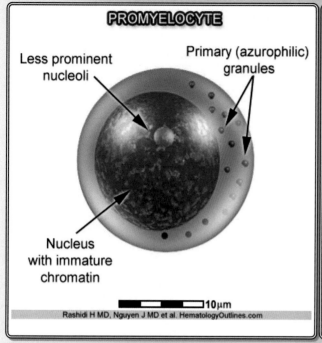

PROMYELOCYTE

Less prominent nucleoli

Primary (azurophilic) granules

Nucleus with immature chromatin

10μm

Rashidi H MD, Nguyen J MD et al. HematologyOutlines.com

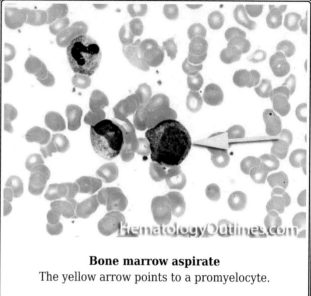

Bone marrow aspirate
The yellow arrow points to a promyelocyte.

🔬 Microscopic Features
- 2-3X larger than a mature RBC
- *High nuclear-to-cytoplasmic ratio (but more cytoplasm than a myeloblast)*
- Round nucleus with immature chromatin (not clumped)
- Nucleoli are present but less prominent than myeloblasts
- Small amount of cytoplasm with primary (azurophilic) granules

⚠ Frequency in Tissues
- Peripheral Blood: ⊘ None
- Bone Marrow: 2-6%
- Lymph Node: ⊘ None

↔ May Resemble
- Myeloblast {p. 21}
- Myelocyte {p. 23}
- Metamyelocyte {p. 24}
- Reactive Lymphocyte {p. 137}
- Neutrophil With Toxic Granules {p. 131}
- Segmented Neutrophil {p. 26}
- Large Granular Lymphocyte {p. 138}

Dx Differential Diagnoses
↑ Increased in:
- ○ Acute promyelocytic leukemia (AKA AML M3)
- ○ Myeloproliferative Neoplasms (e.g. CML)
- ○ Leukemoid reactions
- ○ Post GCSF therapy

⚙ Classic Immunophenotype
- CD34 ⊖
- CD117 ⊕
- HLA-DR ⊖
- CD13 ⊕
- CD33 ⊕
- CD15 ⊖ / ⊕
- MPO ⊕

Miscellaneous: This development stage is the maturation step that comes after myeloblast and precedes myelocyte.

🩸 Myelocyte

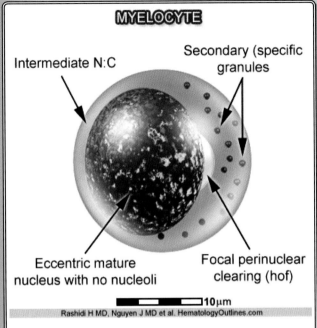

MYELOCYTE

Intermediate N:C

Secondary (specific) granules

Eccentric mature nucleus with no nucleoli

Focal perinuclear clearing (hof)

10 µm

Rashidi H MD, Nguyen J MD et al. HematologyOutlines.com

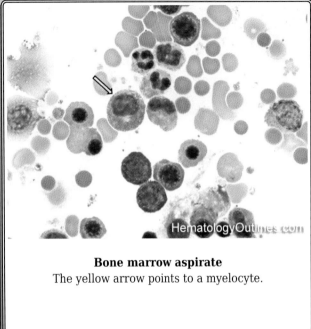

Bone marrow aspirate
The yellow arrow points to a myelocyte.

🔬 Microscopic Features
- 2-3X larger than a mature RBC
- Intermediate nuclear-to-cytoplasmic ratio (more cytoplasm than a promyelocyte)
- *Eccentrically placed oval nucleus (no nucleus indentation) with more mature chromatin (clumped)*
- Perinuclear clearing is common
- Nucleoli are absent (Note: nucleoli are absent from this stage onward)
- More cytoplasm with only rare or absent primary (azurophilic) granules
- Secondary (specific) granules of neutrophilic (lilac), eosinophilic (red-orange), or basophilic (blue) color are present based on precursor type

⚠ Frequency in Tissues
- Peripheral Blood: ⊘ None
- Bone Marrow: ~10%
- Lymph Node: ⊘ None

↔ May Resemble
- Promyelocyte {p. 22}
- Metamyelocyte {p. 24}
- Monocyte {p. 40}
- Reactive Lymphocyte {p. 137}
- Plasma Cell {p. 67}

Ðx Differential Diagnoses
- ↑ Increased in:
  - Chronic myelogenous leukemia (CML)
  - Leukemoid reaction
  - Post GCSF therapy

⚙ Classic Immunophenotype
- CD34 ⊖, HLA-DR ⊖ and CD117 ⊖
- CD13 **dim** ⊞
- CD33 ⊞
- CD15 ⊞
- CD11b ⊞ / ⊖
- CD16 ⊖
- MPO ⊞

Miscellaneous: This is the maturation step that comes after promyelocyte and precedes metamyelocyte.

◊ Metamyelocyte

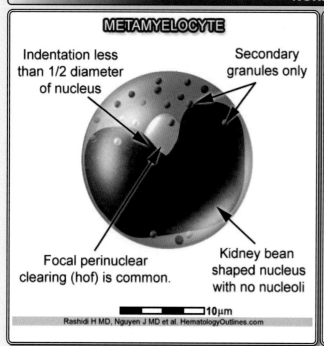

METAMYELOCYTE

Indentation less than 1/2 diameter of nucleus

Secondary granules only

Focal perinuclear clearing (hof) is common.

Kidney bean shaped nucleus with no nucleoli

10µm

Rashidi H MD, Nguyen J MD et al. HematologyOutlines.com

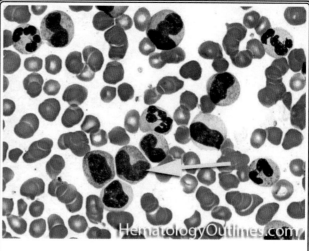

Bone marrow aspirate
The yellow arrow points to a metamyelocyte. Note the nuclear indentation.

🔬 Microscopic Features
- 2-3X larger than a mature RBC
- Intermediate nuclear-to-cytoplasmic (N:C) ratio (more cytoplasm than a promyelocyte)
- *Kidney bean shaped nucleus (indent is less than 1/2 diameter) and mature chromatin (clumped)*
- Perinuclear clearing is common
- Nucleoli are absent
- More cytoplasm with only secondary granules
- Secondary (specific) granules of neutrophilic (lilac), eosinophilic (red-orange), or basophilic (blue) color are present based on precursor type

⚠ Frequency in Tissues
- Peripheral Blood: ⊘ None
- Bone Marrow: ~15%
- Lymph Node: ⊘ None

↔ May Resemble
- Promyelocyte {p. 22}
- Myelocyte {p. 23}
- Band Neutrophil {p. 25}
- Monocyte {p. 40}
- Reactive Lymphocyte {p. 137}
- Mature Segmented Neutrophil {p. 26}

ᴰx Differential Diagnoses
- ↑ Increased in:
  - Chronic myelogenous leukemia (CML)
  - Leukemoid reaction
  - Post GCSF therapy

✪ Classic Immunophenotype
- CD34 ⊖, CD117 ⊖, and HLA-DR ⊖
- CD13 ⊕ and CD33 ⊕
- CD15 ⊕
- CD11b ⊕
- CD16 ⊕
- MPO ⊕

Miscellaneous: This is the maturation step that comes after myelocyte and precedes the band neutrophil.

⬤ Band

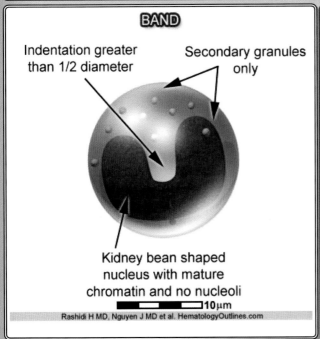

BAND

Indentation greater than 1/2 diameter

Secondary granules only

Kidney bean shaped nucleus with mature chromatin and no nucleoli

⬛⬜⬛⬜10µm

Rashidi H MD, Nguyen J MD et al. HematologyOutlines.com

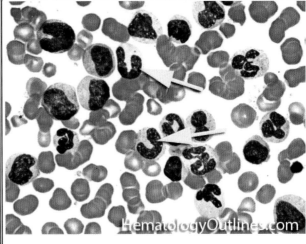

HematologyOutlines.com

Bone marrow aspirate
The yellow arrows point to the band neutrophils.

🔬 Microscopic Features
- 2-3X larger than a mature RBC
- Low nuclear-to-cytoplasmic (N:C) ratio (cytoplasm is relatively increased)
- *Kidney bean-shaped nucleus with indentation (>1/2 the diameter of the nucleus is indented) and mature chromatin (clumped)*
- Nucleoli are absent
- More cytoplasm with only secondary granules
- Secondary (specific) granules of neutrophilic (lilac), eosinophilic (red-orange), or basophilic (blue) color are present based on precursor type

⚠ Frequency in Tissues
- Peripheral Blood: ○ Rare (~1-5%)
- Bone Marrow: ⊗ Scattered (~10-15%)
- Lymph Node: ○ Rare to ⊘ None

↔ May Resemble
- Segmented Neutrophil {p. 26}
- Metamyelocyte {p. 24}
- Myelocyte {p. 23}
- Promyelocyte {p. 22}
- Monocyte {p. 40}

ᴅx Differential Diagnoses
- ↑ Increased in:
  - ○ Infections (especially bacterial)
  - ○ Myeloproliferative disorders (e.g. CML)
  - ○ Leukemoid reaction due to stress, etc.
  - ○ Post-GCSF therapy

⚙ Classic Immunophenotype
- CD34 ⊖, CD117 ⊖, and HLA-DR ⊖
- CD13 ⊞ and CD33 ⊞
- CD15 ⊞
- CD11b ⊞
- CD16 ⊞
- MPO ⊞
- CD10 ⊞ / ⊖

Miscellaneous: When bandemia (increased bands in the peripheral blood) is noted, an underlying infection (especially bacterial) needs to be ruled out.

🔴 Segmented Neutrophil

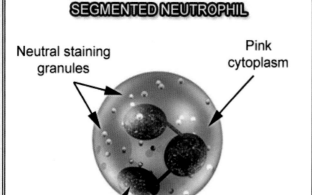

SEGMENTED NEUTROPHIL

Neutral staining granules

Pink cytoplasm

Nucleus with condensed clumped chromatin and 3 to 5 lobes connected by thin chromatin filaments

10μm

Rashidi H MD, Nguyen J MD et al. HematologyOutlines.com

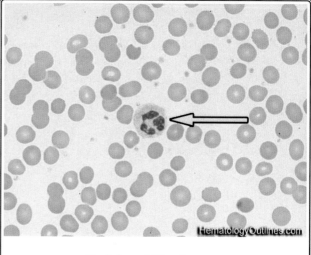

Peripheral blood smear
The yellow arrow points to the segmented neutrophil.

🔬 Microscopic Features
- 2-3X larger than a mature RBC
- Low nuclear-to-cytoplasmic ratio (more cytoplasm than nucleus)
- *Nucleus is mature and divided into 3 to 5 lobes connected by thin chromatin filaments*
- Nucleoli are absent
- More cytoplasm with only secondary granules
- Secondary (specific) granules are neutrophilic (lilac)

⚠️ Frequency in Tissues
- Peripheral Blood: ● Many (most common WBC)
- Bone Marrow: ✪ Scattered
- Lymph Node: ○ Rare to ⊘ None

↔️ May Resemble
- Hypersegmented Neutrophil {p. 130}
- Pseudo-Pelger Huet Neutrophil {p. 132}
- Band Neutrophil {p. 25}
- Neutrophil With Toxic Granules {p. 131}
- Metamyelocyte {p. 24}
- Myelocyte {p. 23}
- Promyelocyte {p. 22}
- Monocyte {p. 40}

ᴰˣ Differential Diagnoses
- ↑ Increased in:
  - ○ Infections (especially bacterial infections)
  - ○ Myeloproliferative disorders (e.g. CML and CNL)
  - ○ Leukemoid reaction
  - ○ Drug-induced

⚙️ Classic Immunophenotype
- CD34 ⊖, CD117 ⊖, and HLA-DR ⊖
- CD10 ⊞, CD13 ⊞ and CD33 ⊞
- CD15 ⊞
- CD11b ⊞
- CD16 ⊞
- MPO ⊞

Miscellaneous: Normal segmentation is 3-5 lobes while hypersegmentation is > 5 lobes and hyposegmentation is < 3 lobes.

⬥ Eosinophil (Precursor)

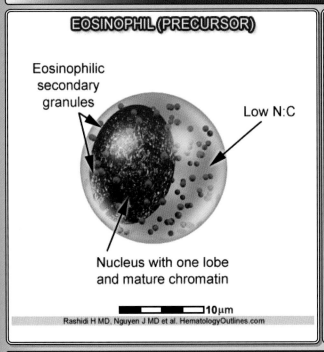

EOSINOPHIL (PRECURSOR)

Eosinophilic secondary granules

Low N:C

Nucleus with one lobe and mature chromatin

▬▬▬▬10µm

Rashidi H MD, Nguyen J MD et al. HematologyOutlines.com

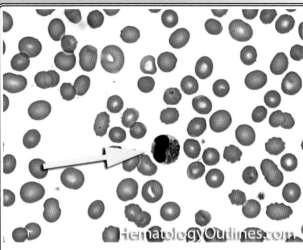

The yellow arrow points to a hypolobated eosinophil precursor.

🔬 Microscopic Features
- 2-3X larger than a mature RBC
- Low nuclear-to-cytoplasmic ratio (more cytoplasm than nucleus)
- ***Nucleus is slightly less mature and usually with 1 lobe***
- Nucleoli may be present depending on stage of maturation
- Secondary (specific) granules are eosinophilic (red-orange) in the myelocyte to mature eosinophil stage

⚠ Frequency in Tissues
- Peripheral Blood: ⊘ None
- Bone Marrow: ○ Rare (~1-2%)
- Lymph Node: ⊘ None

↔ May Resemble
- Mature Eosinophil {p. 28}
- Neutrophilic Myelocyte {p. 23}
- Neutrophilic Metamyelocyte {p. 24}
- Segmented Neutrophil {p. 26}
- Pseudo-Pelger Huet Neutrophil {p. 132}
- Band Neutrophil {p. 25}
- Neutrophil With Toxic Granules {p. 131}
- Promyelocyte {p. 22}
- Basophil {p. 29}

Dx Differential Diagnoses
- ↑ Increased in:
  - Myeloproliferative neoplasms (some)
  - Allergy-related (e.g. Asthma)
  - Drug reactions
  - Invasive parasitic infections
  - Acute myeloid leukemia (rare variants)

⚙ Classic Immunophenotype
- N/A

Miscellaneous: Hypolobation of the precursor eosinophil is due to its immaturity.

🩸 Eosinophil (Mature)

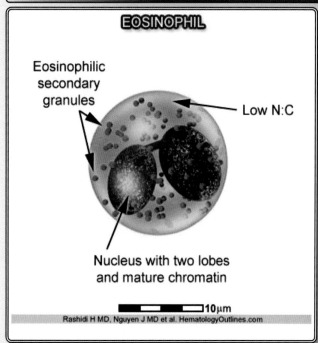

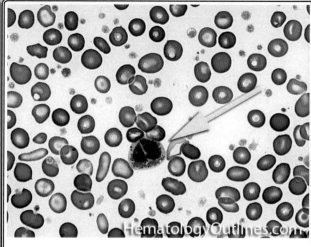

The arrow points to the mature eosinophil. Note the bilobed nucleus and prominent red granules.

🔬 Microscopic Features
- 2-3X larger than a mature RBC
- Low nuclear-to-cytoplasmic ratio (more cytoplasm than nucleus)
- *Nucleus is mature and usually with 2 lobes connected by thin chromatin filament*
- Nucleoli are absent
- More cytoplasm with only secondary granules
- *Secondary (specific) granules are eosinophilic (red-orange color)*

⚠ Frequency in Tissues
- Peripheral Blood: ✺ Scattered (4th most common WBC in blood, after neutrophils, lymphocytes and monocytes)
- Bone Marrow: ○ Rare
- Lymph Node: ○ Rare to ⊘ None

↔ May Resemble
- Segmented Neutrophil {p. 26}
- Pseudo-Pelger Huet Neutrophil {p. 132}
- Band Neutrophil {p. 25}
- Neutrophil With Toxic Granules {p. 131}
- Promyelocyte {p. 22}
- Basophil {p. 29}

ᴰˣ Differential Diagnoses
- ↑ Increased in:
  - Allergy-related (e.g. Asthma)
  - Drug reactions
  - Invasive parasitic infections
  - Myeloproliferative neoplasms
  - Hodgkin's and non-Hodgkin's lymphomas
  - Autoimmune disorders (some)

⚙ Classic Immunophenotype
- CD45 **dim** ➕
- CD10 ➖, CD14 ➖, CD64 ➖, HLA-DR ➖
- High SSC (side light scatter)
- CD13 **dim** ➕, CD33 ➕, CD11b ➕, CD11c ➕
- CD16 ➖
- CD15 **dim** ➕

Miscellaneous: Increased amounts are commonly associated with: drugs, allergy, infection (especially invasive multicellular parasites), neoplasms (e.g. myeloid neoplasms such as some AMLs or MPNs), and idiopathic causes.

🔴 Basophil (Mature)

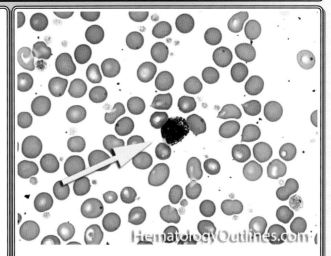

BASOPHIL

Mature nucleus has 2-3 lobes

Low N:C

Nucleus may be obscured by numerous basophilic secondary granules

10μm

Rashidi H MD, Nguyen J MD et al. HematologyOutlines.com

The arrow points to the basophil. Notice the granules obscuring the nucleus.

🔬 Microscopic Features
- 2-3X larger than a mature RBC
- Low nuclear-to-cytoplasmic ratio (more cytoplasm than nucleus)
- Nucleus is mature and usually with 2-3 lobes connected by a thin chromatin filament
- Nucleoli are absent and more cytoplasm with only secondary granules
- *Secondary (specific) granules are basophilic (blue-violet color) and obscure the underlying nucleus*

⚠ Frequency in Tissues
- Peripheral Blood: ○ Rare (5th most common WBC)
- Bone Marrow: ○ Rare
- Lymph Node: ⊘ None

↔ May Resemble
- Eosinophil {p. 28}
- Segmented Neutrophil {p. 26}
- Pseudo-Pelger Huet Neutrophil {p. 132}
- Neutrophil With Toxic Granules {p. 131}
- Promyelocyte {p. 22}
- Mast cell (see in Glossary)

℞x Differential Diagnoses
- CML accelerated phase AML (rare variants)
- Infection (e.g. varicella)
- Hypersensitivity reactions

⚙ Classic Immunophenotype
- CD34 ⊖ and CD117 ⊖
- CD45 **dim** ⊕ (less bright than lymphocytes)
- Low SSC (side light scatter)
- CD11b ⊕ and CD13 ⊕
- CD22 ⊕, CD25 **dim** ⊕, CD33 ⊕
- CD38 ⊕⊕ and CD123 ⊕⊕
- CD16 ⊖ and CD15 ⊖

Miscellaneous: Increased basophils may be associated with some myeloid neoplasms such as CML, some infections or some hypersensitivity reactions. Basophils and mast cells are distinct from one another but share some similar morphologic and functional aspects. As opposed to basophils which can be seen in the peripheral blood, mast cells are only seen in tissue and absent from the peripheral blood. Additionally, the nucleus of the mast cell is usually round and not segmented as opposed to the basophil's segmented (usually bi-lobed) nucleus. The granules of basophils are more heterogenous and overlap the nucleus while the granules of mast cells are more uniform and less often cover the nucleus.

⬥ Pseudo Pelger Huet Neutrophil

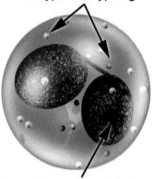

PSEUDO PELGER-HUET NEUTROPHIL

Lack of normal cytoplasmic granules
(sometimes hypo- or hyper-granulation)

Irregular nuclear lobation
(usually hypolobated)

⬛⬜⬛⬜**10µm**

Rashidi H MD, Nguyen J MD et al. HematologyOutlines.com

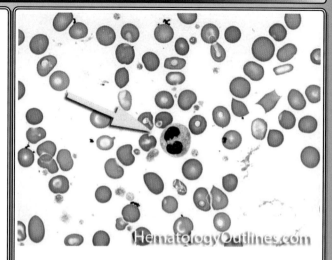

The yellow arrow points to the bilobed pseudo Pelger
Huet neutrophil (2 lobes, instead of the normal 3-5
lobes)

🔬 Microscopic Features
- 2-3X larger than a mature RBC
- Low nuclear-to-cytoplasmic ratio (more cytoplasm than nucleus)
- *Nucleus is mature with 2 lobes connected by a thin chromatin filament*
- Nucleoli are absent
- In some cases, hypergranulation, hypogranulation or abnormal granules can be seen
- Pseudo Pelger-Huet neutrophils are a form of dysplastic neutrophils
- In younger patients these cells may represent Pelger Huet anomaly

⚠ Frequency in Tissues
- Peripheral Blood: ○ Rare to ⊘ None
- Bone Marrow: ○ Rare to ⊘ None
- Lymph Node: ⊘ None

↔ May Resemble
- Eosinophil {p. 28}
- Segmented Neutrophil {p. 26}
- Band Neutrophil {p. 25}
- Neutrophil With Toxic Granules {p. 131}
- Basophil {p. 29}

ᴅx Differential Diagnoses
- Myelodysplastic syndrome (MDS)
- Pelger Huet anomaly (if they are true Pelger Huet cells)

⚙ Classic Immunophenotype
- CD45 ➕
- Lowered SCC (side scatter)
- CD10 ➖ / ➕
- CD11b ➕ / ➖
- CD13 ➕ / ➖
- CD16 ➕ / ➖

Miscellaneous: Normal segmentation is 3-5 lobes while hyposegmentation is < 3 lobes and hypersegmentation is > 5 lobes. The immunoprofile may be aberrant if it is dysplastic and associated with myelodysplastic syndrome (MDS).

🔻 Hypogranular or Agranular Neutrophil

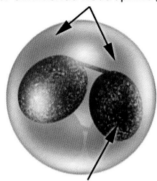

HYPOGRANULAR OR AGRANULAR NEUTROPHIL

Lack or diminished neutrophilic granules

Mature nucleus with two lobes connected by thin chromatin filament

■■■■■■10μm

Rashidi H MD, Nguyen J MD et al. HematologyOutlines.com

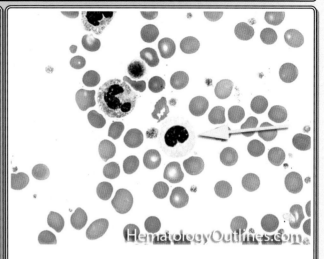

The yellow arrow points to the hypogranular (lack of granules) band neutrophil.

🔬 Microscopic Features
- 2-3X larger than a mature RBC
- Low nuclear-to-cytoplasmic ratio (more cytoplasm than nucleus)
- Nucleus is mature
- Nucleoli are absent
- *Lack or diminished neutrophilic granules*

⚠ Frequency in Tissues
- Peripheral Blood: ◯ Rare to ⊘ None
- Bone Marrow: ◯ Rare to ⊘ None
- Lymph Node: ⊘ None

↔ May Resemble
- Segmented Neutrophil {p. 26}
- Band Neutrophil {p. 25}
- Monocyte {p. 40}

℞x Differential Diagnoses
- Myelodysplastic syndrome (MDS)
- Staining artifact giving rise to pseudo-hypogranularity

⚙ Classic Immunophenotype
- CD45 ⊞
- Lowered SCC (side scatter)
- CD10 ⊖ / ⊞
- CD11b ⊞ / ⊖
- CD13 ⊞ / ⊖
- CD16 ⊞ / ⊖

Miscellaneous: The low side scatter (SCC) noted in flow cytometry is due to the hypogranularity. The immunoprofile may be aberrant if it is dysplastic and associated with myelodysplastic syndrome (MDS).

Myeloblast with Auer Rod

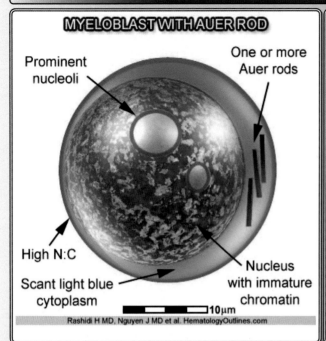

MYELOBLAST WITH AUER ROD

Prominent nucleoli

One or more Auer rods

High N:C

Scant light blue cytoplasm

Nucleus with immature chromatin

10μm

Rashidi H MD, Nguyen J MD et al. HematologyOutlines.com

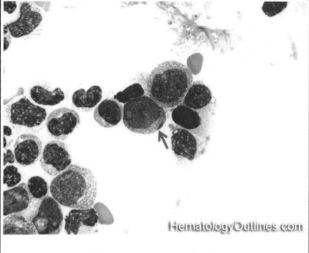

Bone marrow aspirate
The red arrow is pointing to the Auer rod in the abnormal myeloblast.

🔬 Microscopic Features
- 3-4X larger than a mature RBC
- *High nuclear-to-cytoplasmic (N:C) ratio*
- Round nucleus with immature chromatin (not clumped)
- Prominent nucleoli
- Cytoplasm is scant, gray to pale blue and usually lacks granules
- One or more red-pink rod shaped structures called Auer rod(s) are noted in the cytoplasm

⚠ Frequency in Tissues
- Peripheral Blood: ⊘ None
- Bone Marrow: ⊘ None
- Lymph Node: ⊘ None

↔ May Resemble
- Promyelocyte {p. 22}
- Pronormoblast {p. 9}
- Lymphoblast {p. 65}
- Monoblast {p. 38}
- Reactive Lymphocyte {p. 137}

ᴅx Differential Diagnoses
- Acute myeloid leukemia (AML)
- Myelodysplastic syndromes (specifically RAEB-2, now known as MDS with excess blasts-2)

⚙ Classic Immunophenotype
- CD34 ⊞
- CD117 ⊞
- HLA-DR ⊞
- CD13 ⊞
- CD33 ⊞
- May also have immunophenotypic aberrancies such as gain of CD56 or CD7, etc.

Miscellaneous: The presence of an Auer rod(s) is diagnostic of the myeloid origin of the blast cell (the only morphologic feature that could reliably distinguish a myeloblast from a lymphoblast).

♩**Note**: Other types of blasts (e.g. lymphoblasts) lack Auer rods.

🔴 Promyelocyte with Auer Rods

PROMYELOCYTE WITH AUER RODS

Prominent nucleoli

Primary (azurophilic) granules

Nucleus with immature chromatin

Multiple Auer rods may be seen

10µm

Rashidi H MD, Nguyen J MD et al. HematologyOutlines.com

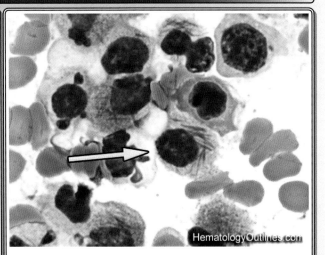

Bone marrow aspirate
The yellow arrow points to an abnormal promyelocyte with multiple Auer rods.

🔬 Microscopic Features
- 3-4X larger than a mature RBC
- High nuclear-to-cytoplasmic (N:C) ratio
- *Round nucleus with immature chromatin (not clumped)*
- Prominent nucleoli
- Cytoplasm is not as scant as a myeloblast, gray to pale blue with primary granules
- Multiple Auer rods may be seen as well

⚠ Frequency in Tissues
- Peripheral Blood: ⊘ None
- Bone Marrow: ⊘ None
- Lymph Node: ⊘ None

↔ May Resemble
- Myeloblast {p. 21}
- Pronormoblast {p. 9}
- Lymphoblast {p. 65}
- Monoblast {p. 38}
- Reactive Lymphocyte {p. 137}
- Rarely may represent other AMLs

ᴅx Differential Diagnoses
- If seen in the peripheral blood or in the bone marrow, then must rule out an acute promyelocytic leukemia (APL).
- Other AMLs

⚙ Classic Immunophenotype
- CD34 ⊖
- CD117 ⊞
- HLA-DR ⊖
- CD11c ⊖
- CD13 ⊞
- CD33 ⊞
- May also have immunophenotypic aberrancies such as gain of CD56, etc.

Miscellaneous: A promyelocyte with multiple Auer rods may resemble a "bundle of sticks," as the numerous Auer rods resemble it.

♦ Eosinophil (Increased)

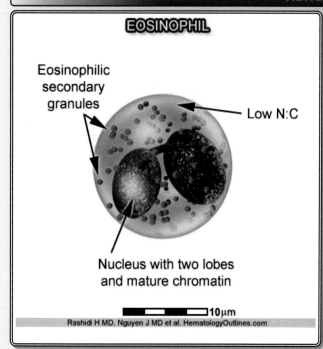

EOSINOPHIL

Eosinophilic secondary granules

Low N:C

Nucleus with two lobes and mature chromatin

10μm

Rashidi H MD, Nguyen J MD et al. HematologyOutlines.com

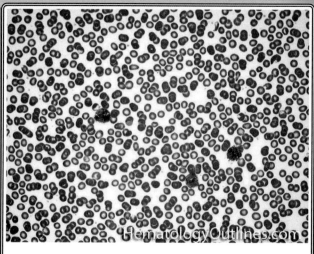

Three eosinophils are seen among many red blood cells.

🔬 Microscopic Features
- 2-3X larger than a mature RBC
- Low nuclear-to-cytoplasmic ratio (more cytoplasm than nucleus)
- *Nucleus is mature and usually with 2 lobes connected by thin chromatin filament*
- Nucleoli are absent
- More cytoplasm with only secondary granules
- *Secondary (specific) granules are eosinophilic (red-orange color)*

⚠ Frequency in Tissues
- Peripheral Blood: ✳ Scattered (4th most common WBC in blood, after neutrophils, lymphocytes and monocytes)
- Bone Marrow: ○ Rare
- Lymph Node: ○ Rare to ⊘ None

↔ May Resemble
- Segmented Neutrophil {p. 26}
- Pseudo-Pelger Huet Neutrophil {p. 132}
- Band Neutrophil {p. 25}
- Neutrophil With Toxic Granules {p. 131}
- Promyelocyte {p. 22}
- Basophil {p. 29}

ᴰx Differential Diagnoses
- Allergy-related (e.g. Asthma)
- Drug reactions
- Invasive parasitic infections
- Myeloproliferative neoplasms
- Hodgkin's and non-Hodgkin's lymphomas
- Autoimmune disorders (some)

⚙ Classic Immunophenotype
- CD45 **dim** ➕
- HLA-DR ➖, CD10 ➖
- CD14 ➖, CD64 ➖
- High SSC (Side light scatter)
- CD13 **dim** ➕, CD15 **dim** ➕, CD33 ➕
- CD11b ➕, CD11c ➕
- CD16 ➖

Miscellaneous: Increased amounts are commonly associated with: drugs, allergy, infection (specially invasive multicellular parasites), neoplasms (e.g. myeloid neoplasms such as some AMLs or MPNs), and idiopathic.

🔹 Dysplastic Eosinophil

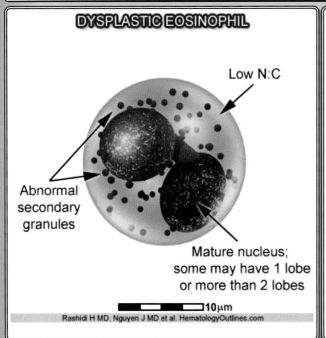

DYSPLASTIC EOSINOPHIL

Low N:C

Abnormal secondary granules

Mature nucleus; some may have 1 lobe or more than 2 lobes

10µm

Rashidi H MD, Nguyen J MD et al. HematologyOutlines.com

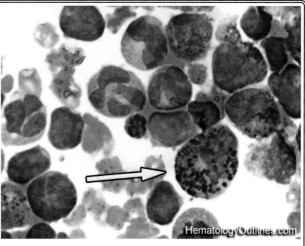

Bone marrow aspirate
The yellow arrow points to an abnormal eosinophil with abnormal basophilic-like granules.

🔬 Microscopic Features
- 2-3X larger than a mature RBC
- Low nuclear-to-cytoplasmic ratio (more cytoplasm than nucleus)
- Nucleus is mature and usually with 2 lobes connected by thin chromatin (some have 1 lobe or > 2 lobes)
- Nucleoli are absent
- *More cytoplasm with abnormal secondary granules (usually darker in color like basophilic granules)*
- The granules are heterogenous and vacuoules may occasionally be noted as well

⚠ Frequency in Tissues
- Peripheral Blood: ⊘ None
- Bone Marrow: ⊘ None
- Lymph Node: ⊘ None

↔ May Resemble
- Eosinophil {p. 28}
- Basophil {p. 29}
- Neutrophil (mature) {p. 26}
- Pseudo-Pelger Huet Neutrophil {p. 132}
- Band Neutrophil {p. 25}

ᴰx Differential Diagnoses
- Certain AMLs such as AML with inv 16 or t(16;16) (aka M4Eo)
- Certain myeloproliferative neoplasms
- Certain myelodysplastic syndromes (MDS)

⚙ Classic Immunophenotype
- CD45 **dim** ➕ with high SSC (side light scatter)
- CD13 **dim** ➕
- CD16 ➖
- CD15 **dim** ➕
- May have some immunophenotypic variability compared to normal eosinophils

Miscellaneous: AML with inv16 or t(16;16) was also known as AML-M4Eo (which defined an AML with monocytic differentiation and abnormal eosinophils). The gene involved is CBF-B.

🩸 Basophils (Increased)

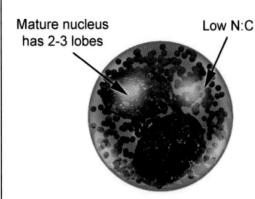

BASOPHIL

Mature nucleus has 2-3 lobes

Low N:C

Nucleus may be obscured by numerous basophilic secondary granules

10μm

Rashidi H MD, Nguyen J MD et al. HematologyOutlines.com

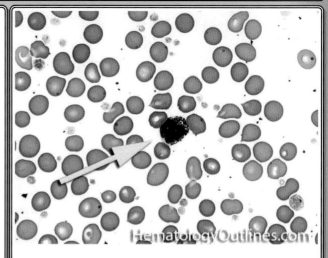

The yellow arrow points to a basophil. Basophils are rarely seen in a normal blood smear.

🔬 Microscopic Features
- 2-3X larger than a mature RBC
- Low nuclear-to-cytoplasmic ratio (more cytoplasm than nucleus)
- Nucleus is mature and usually with 2-3 lobes connected by a thin chromatin filament
- Nucleoli are absent
- More cytoplasm with only secondary granules
- *Secondary (specific) granules are basophilic (blue-violet color) and obscure the underlying nucleus*

⚠ Frequency in Tissues
- Peripheral Blood: Very Rare (5th most common WBC in blood, after neutrophils, lymphocytes, monocytes, and Eosinophils)
- Bone Marrow: ○ Rare
- Lymph Node: ⊘ None

↔ May Resemble
- Eosinophil {p. 28}
- Segmented Neutrophil {p. 26}
- Pseudo-Pelger Huet Neutrophil {p. 132}
- Band Neutrophil {p. 25}
- Neutrophil With Toxic Granules {p. 131}
- Promyelocyte {p. 22}
- Mast cell (see in Glossary)

ᴅx Differential Diagnoses
- CML accelerated phase
- AML (rare variants)
- Infection (e.g. varicella)
- Hypersensitivity reactions (sometimes)

⚙ Classic Immunophenotype
- CD34 ⊖ and CD117 ⊖
- CD45 **dim** ⊞ (less bright than lymphocytes)
- Low SSC (side light scatter)
- CD11b ⊞ and CD13 ⊞
- CD22 ⊞, CD25 **dim** ⊞, CD33 ⊞
- CD38 ⊞⊞ and CD123 ⊞⊞
- CD16 ⊖ and CD15 ⊖

Miscellaneous: Increased basophils may be associated with some myeloid neoplasms such as CML, some infections, or sometimes in hypersensitivity reactions.

Monocyte Maturation Overview Diagram

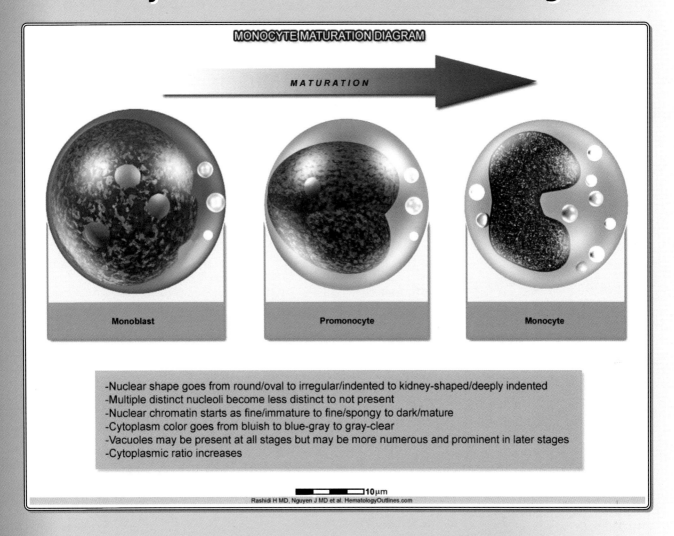

MONOCYTE MATURATION DIAGRAM

MATURATION

Monoblast **Promonocyte** **Monocyte**

-Nuclear shape goes from round/oval to irregular/indented to kidney-shaped/deeply indented
-Multiple distinct nucleoli become less distinct to not present
-Nuclear chromatin starts as fine/immature to fine/spongy to dark/mature
-Cytoplasm color goes from bluish to blue-gray to gray-clear
-Vacuoles may be present at all stages but may be more numerous and prominent in later stages
-Cytoplasmic ratio increases

10μm

Rashidi H MD, Nguyen J MD et al. HematologyOutlines.com

Stages of maturation go from monoblast to promonocyte to monocyte to macrophage. The nucleus is oval, horseshoe or kidney shaped and is usually eccentric. The chromatin is less dense than in lymphocytes.

Monoblasts and promonocytes are rare and predominantly contained to the bone marrow while mature monocytes are mostly seen in peripheral blood. As mature monocytes leave the peripheral blood and enter tissue, they become macrophages/histiocytes.

Monoblasts and promonocytes contain nucleoli (a sign of immaturity), while the mature monocytes and macrophages lack nucleoli (since they are mature).

◊ Monoblast

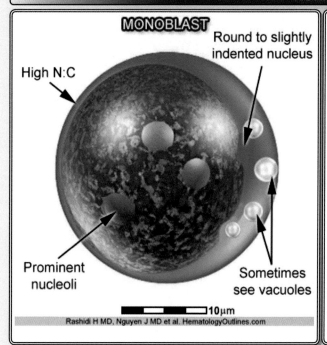

MONOBLAST

High N:C

Round to slightly indented nucleus

Prominent nucleoli

Sometimes see vacuoles

10μm

Rashidi H MD, Nguyen J MD et al. HematologyOutlines.com

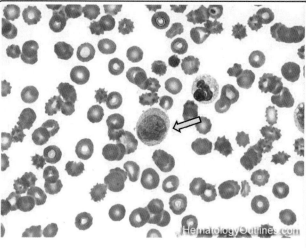

The arrow points to the monoblast. Notice the round nucleus and the prominent nucleolus.

🔬 Microscopic Features

- 3-4X larger than a mature RBC
- *High nuclear-to-cytoplasmic ratio*
- Round to slightly indented nucleus with immature chromatin (not clumped)
- Prominent nucleoli
- Cytoplasm is scant, gray to pale blue (more cytoplasm than a myeloblast and with rare or absent granules)
- Vacuoles are rare but sometimes noted in cytoplasm

⚠ Frequency in Tissues

- Peripheral Blood: ⊘ None
- Bone Marrow: 1%
- Lymph Node: ⊘ None

↔ May Resemble

- Promonocyte {p. 39}
- Myeloblast {p. 21}
- Lymphoblast {p. 65}
- Pronormoblast {p. 9}
- Mature Monocyte {p. 40}
- Reactive Lymphocyte {p. 137}
- Lymphoma cell (e.g. Leukemic phase of Burkitt lymphoma)
- Metastic carcinoma cell

ᴅx Differential Diagnoses

↑ Increased in:
- ○ Acute monocytic leukemia (AML)
- ○ Acute myelomonocytic leukemia (AMML)
- ○ Chronic myelomonocytic leukemia (CMML)

⚙ Classic Immunophenotype

- CD34 ⊞ / ⊟, CD117 ⊞ / ⊟
- HLA-DR ⊞
- CD13 ⊞ and CD33 ⊞
- CD64 ⊞
- CD4 **dim** ⊞
- CD14 ⊟

Miscellaneous: In monocyte-differentiated leukemias, the total blast count is equal to monoblasts + promonocytes (since promonocytes are considered in this instance to be equivalent to blasts).

◊ Promonocyte

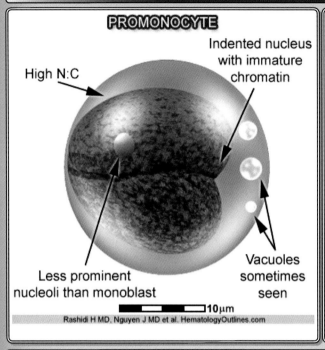

PROMONOCYTE

High N:C

Indented nucleus with immature chromatin

Less prominent nucleoli than monoblast

Vacuoles sometimes seen

10μm

Rashidi H MD, Nguyen J MD et al. HematologyOutlines.com

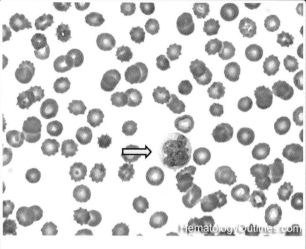

The yellow arrow points to the promonocyte. Note the prominent nucleolus.

🔬 Microscopic Features
- 3-4X larger than a mature RBC
- *Round indented nucleus with immature chromatin (not clumped; slightly more mature than monoblast)*
- Prominent nucleoli (less prominent than monoblast)
- Cytoplasm is scant but more than myeloblasts, gray to pale blue and with rare or no granules
- Vacuoles are maybe sometimes noted in the cytoplasm

⚠ Frequency in Tissues
- Peripheral Blood: ⊘ None
- Bone Marrow: 1%
- Lymph Node: ⊘ None

↔ May Resemble
- Monoblast {p. 38}
- Myeloblast {p. 21}
- Mature Monocyte {p. 40}
- Reactive Lymphocyte {p. 137}
- Lymphoma cell (e.g. Leukemic phase of Burkitt lymphoma)
- Metastatic carcinoma cell

℞ Differential Diagnoses
- ↑ Increased in:
  - Acute monocytic leukemia (AML)
  - Acute myelomonocytic leukemia (AMML)
  - Chronic myelomonocytic leukemia (CMML)
- Infection/inflammation

⚙ Classic Immunophenotype
- CD34 ⊖, CD117 ⊖/⊕, HLA-DR ⊕
- CD13 ⊕, CD15 ⊕, CD33 ⊕
- CD64 ⊕
- CD14 ⊖/⊕
- CD4 **dim** ⊕

Miscellaneous: Promonocytes count as blasts when accounting for the total blast count. In myeloid leukemias with monocytic differentiation, the total blast count is equal to monoblasts + promonocytes.

◊ Monocyte

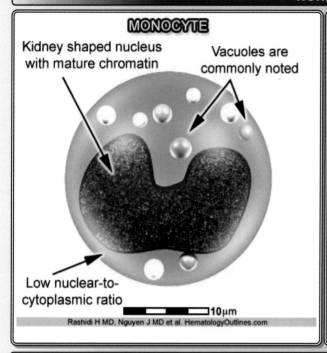

MONOCYTE

Kidney shaped nucleus with mature chromatin

Vacuoles are commonly noted

Low nuclear-to-cytoplasmic ratio

10μm

Rashidi H MD, Nguyen J MD et al. HematologyOutlines.com

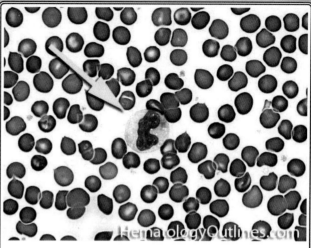

The yellow arrow points to the mature monocyte. Notice the kidney shaped nucleus and cytoplasmic vacuoles.

🔬 Microscopic Features
- 3-4X larger than a mature RBC
- Lower nuclear-to-cytoplasmic ratio because of increased cytoplasm
- *Kidney-shaped indented nucleus with mature chromatin (clumped)*
- Nucleoli are absent
- Cytoplasm is abundant, gray to pale blue and with rare to no granules
- Vacuoles are commonly noted in cytoplasm

⚠ Frequency in Tissues
- Peripheral Blood: 3rd most common WBC (after neutrophils and lymphocytes)
- Bone Marrow: ✺ Scattered (some in the form of histiocytes/macrophages)
- Lymph Node: ✺ Scattered (some in the form of histiocytes/macrophages)

↔ May Resemble
- Reactive Lymphocyte {p. 137}
- Myelocyte {p. 23}
- Metamyelocyte {p. 24}
- Band Neutrophil {p. 25}
- Promonocyte {p. 39}
- Monoblast {p. 38}

Ⓓx Differential Diagnoses
- ↑ Increased in:
  - ○ Chronic myelomonocytic leukemia (CMML)
  - ○ Autoimmune disorders (sometimes)
  - ○ Chronic infections (e.g. CMV, tuberculosis, etc.)

⚙ Classic Immunophenotype
- CD45 ⊞
- CD34 ⊖, CD1147 ⊖, and HLA-DR ⊞
- Intermediate SSC (side light scatter)
- CD14 ⊞ and CD64 ⊞
- CD13 ⊞, CD15 ⊞, and CD33 ⊞
- CD4 **dim** ⊞

Miscellaneous: Monocytes leave the peripheral blood and enter tissue to become macrophages/histiocytes. In contraast to monoblasts and promonocytes (which have nucleoli), mature monocytes and macrophages/histiocytes lack nucleoli.

🌢 Increased Mature Monocytes

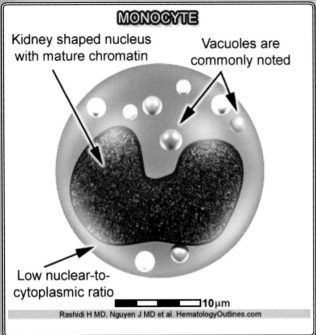

MONOCYTE

Kidney shaped nucleus with mature chromatin

Vacuoles are commonly noted

Low nuclear-to-cytoplasmic ratio

10μm

Rashidi H MD, Nguyen J MD et al. HematologyOutlines.com

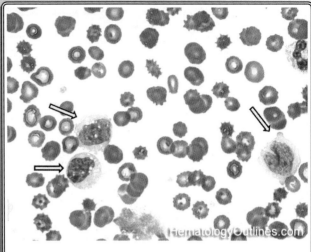

The yellow arrows point out the increase in monocytes in the field of view. Notice the lack of a nucleolus in these mature monocytes.

🔬 Microscopic Features
- 3-4X larger than a mature RBC
- Lower nuclear-to-cytoplasmic ratio because of increased cytoplasm
- *Kidney-shaped indented nucleus with mature chromatin (clumped)*
- Nucleoli is absent cytoplasm is abundant, gray to pale blue and lacks granules
- Vacuoles are commonly noted in cytoplasm

⚠ Frequency in Tissues
- Peripheral Blood: 3rd most common WBC (after neutrophils and lymphocytes)
- Bone Marrow: ⚽ Scattered (some as histiocytes/macrophages)
- Lymph Node: ⚽ Scattered (some as histiocytes/macrophages)

↔ May Resemble
- Reactive Lymphocyte {p. 137}
- Myelocyte {p. 23}
- Metamyelocyte {p. 24}
- Band Neutrophil {p. 25}
- Promonocyte {p. 39}
- Monoblast {p. 38}

Dx Differential Diagnoses
- Chronic myelomonocytic leukemia (CMML)
- Chronic neutropenia
- Autoimmune (sometimes)
- Chronic infections (e.g. CMV, tuberculosis, etc.)

⚙ Classic Immunophenotype
- CD45 ➕
- CD34 ➖, CD1147 ➖, and HLA-DR ➕
- Intermediate SSC (side light scatter)
- CD14 ➕ and CD64 ➕
- CD13 ➕, CD15 ➕, and CD33 ➕
- CD4 **dim** ➕

Miscellaneous: Increased monocytes can be associated with many processes including but not limited to infectious etiologies, myeloproliferative neoplasms (e.g. CML), MPN/MDS (e.g. CMML), etc.

♦ Histoplasmosis in Histiocytes

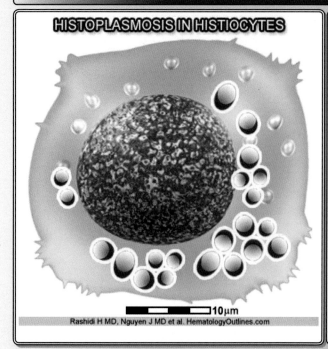

HISTOPLASMOSIS IN HISTIOCYTES

10μm

Rashidi H MD, Nguyen J MD et al. HematologyOutlines.com

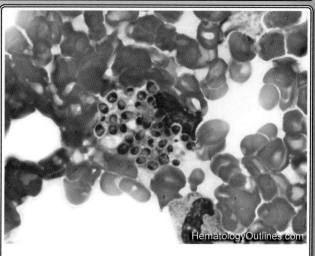

HematologyOutlines.com

The center of the image is a monocyte packed with histoplasmosis.

☌ Microscopic Features
- *Small round fungal forms seen within the cytoplasm of mature monocytes and histiocytes*

⚠ Frequency in Tissues
- Peripheral Blood: ⊘ None
- Bone Marrow: ⊘ None
- Lymph Node: ⊘ None

↔ May Resemble
- Leishmania In Histiocytes {p. 43}
- Cellular debris in histiocytes
- Bacteria in histiocytes

ᴅx Differential Diagnoses
- Histoplasmosis
- Leishmaniasis
- Cellular debris within histiocytes
- Bacterial infection

⚙ Classic Immunophenotype
- N/A

Miscellaneous: Histoplasma fungal forms lack kinetoplasts (small dark blue rod shaped structures within the organism) which are present in leishmania (a parasite that may resemble histoplasma).

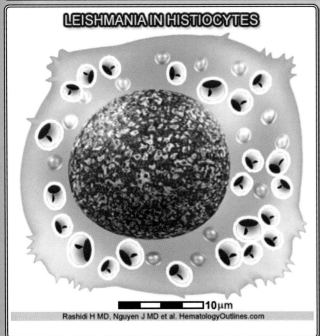

LEISHMANIA IN HISTIOCYTES

10μm

Rashidi H MD, Nguyen J MD et al. HematologyOutlines.com

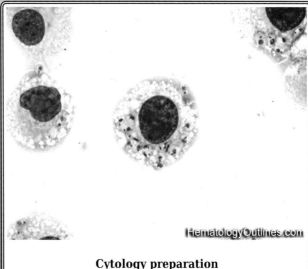

HematologyOutlines.com

Cytology preparation
Note the macrophages with multiple leishmania parasites.

🔬 Microscopic Features
- *Small round/oval parasitic forms with kinetoplasts are noted here within the cytoplasm of this histiocyte*

⚠ Frequency in Tissues
- Peripheral Blood: ⊘ None
- Bone Marrow: ⊘ None
- Lymph Node: ⊘ None

↔ May Resemble
- Histoplasma In Histiocytes {p. 42}
- Cellular debris in histiocytes
- Bacteria in histiocytes

ᴰx Differential Diagnoses
- Leishmaniasis
- Histoplasmosis
- Cellular debris within histiocytes
- Bacterial infection

⚙ Classic Immunophenotype
- N/A

Miscellaneous: Histoplasma fungal forms lack kinetoplasts (small dark blue rod shaped structures within the organism) which are present in leishmania, but absent in histoplasma.

⬦ Mycobacteria in Histiocytes

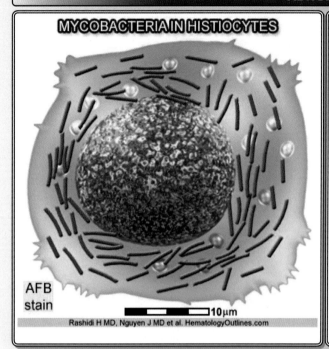

MYCOBACTERIA IN HISTIOCYTES

AFB stain

⊢━━━━━⊣10µm

Rashidi H MD, Nguyen J MD et al. HematologyOutlines.com

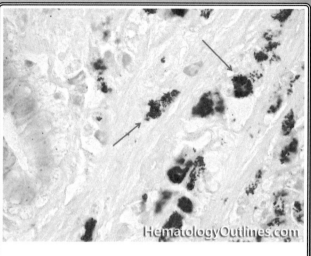

HematologyOutlines.com

Acid-fast stain
The acid-fast stain highlights numerous red rod shaped organisms within the cytoplasm of the histiocytes.

🔬 Microscopic Features
- *Rod shaped acid fast bacilli present in the cytoplasm of histiocytes*
- Acid-fast stain highlights them as red rod shaped small structures

⚠ Frequency in Tissues
- Peripheral Blood: ⊘ None
- Bone Marrow: ⊘ None
- Lymph Node: ⊘ None

⟷ May Resemble
- Histoplasma In Histiocytes {p. 42}
- Leishmania In Histiocytes {p. 43}
- Cellular debris in histiocytes
- Bacteria in histiocytes

ᴰx Differential Diagnoses
- Leishmaniasis
- Histoplasmosis
- Cellular debris within histiocytes
- Bacterial infection
- Mycobacterium avium intracellulaire
- Mycobacterium leprae
- Mycobacterium tuberculosis

⚙ Classic Immunophenotype
- N/A

Miscellaneous: Mycobacteria are usually acid-fast stain positive. These can be of a variety of species such as M. tuberculosis (in which acid fast bacilli organisms are rare and not easily identified) or M. leprae and MAI (in which acid fast bacilli may be plenty and readily seen with special stain).

Megakarocyte Maturation Overview Diagram

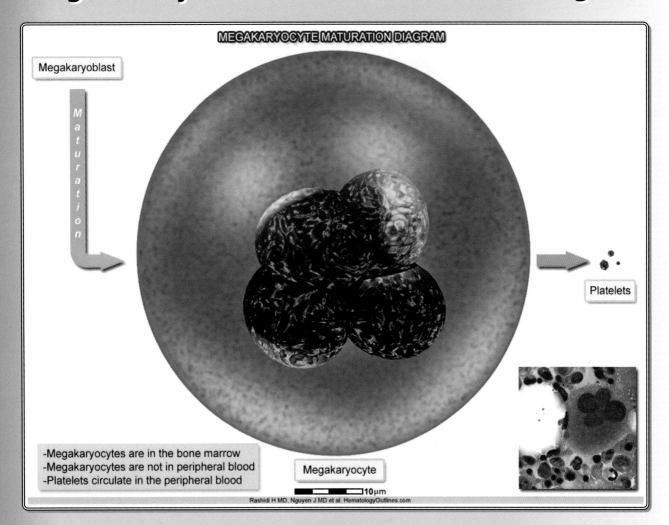

MEGAKARYOCYTE MATURATION DIAGRAM

Megakaryoblast

Maturation

Platelets

Megakaryocyte

-Megakaryocytes are in the bone marrow
-Megakaryocytes are not in peripheral blood
-Platelets circulate in the peripheral blood

10μm

Rashidi H MD, Nguyen J MD et al. HematologyOutlines.com

Megakaryocytes are the largest bone marrow cells with a dark, multilobulated nucleus and are responsible for the production of platelets. Their nucleus multiplies but without cellular cytoplasmic division. Hence they can end up having increased numbers of chromatin (typically 4N). Megakaryocytes are stimulated by thrombopoietin (TPO) which enables their maturation and ultimately allowing them to increase platelet production. These platelets are derived from cytoplasmic projections of megakaryocytes which play a central role in hemostasis.

🌢 Megakaryocyte

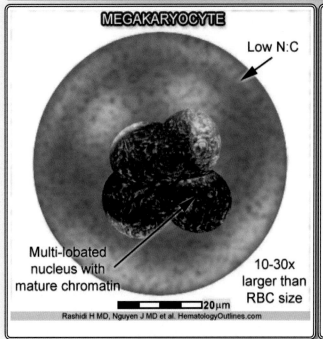

MEGAKARYOCYTE

Low N:C

Multi-lobated nucleus with mature chromatin

10-30x larger than RBC size

20μm

Rashidi H MD, Nguyen J MD et al. HematologyOutlines.com

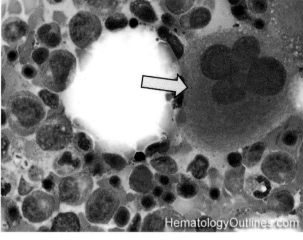

Bone marrow aspirate
The arrow points to the megakaryocyte. Note its size difference compared to the surrounding cells.

🔬 Microscopic Features
- 10-30X larger than a mature RBC (largest hematopoietic cell)
- Lower nuclear-to-cytoplasmic ratio because of increased cytoplasm
- *Multilobated nucleus (2-8 lobes on top of each other) with mature chromatin (clumped)*
- Nucleoli are absent
- Cytoplasm is abundant and light blue and usually lacks granules

⚠ Frequency in Tissues
- Peripheral Blood: ⊘ None
- Bone Marrow: ✦ Scattered
- Lymph Node: ⊘ None
- May be seen in spleen and liver of newborns or those with extramedullary hematopoiesis

↔ May Resemble
- Osteoclasts
- Histiocytes and macrophages (especially multinucleated forms)
- Hodgkin Lymphoma Reed Sternberg cell (see in Glossary)
- Metastatic tumor cells

℞x Differential Diagnoses
- Peripheral destruction of platelets (e.g. ITP) may lead to megakaryocytic hyperplasia in the marrow
- Myeloproliferative neoplasms
- Myelodysplastic syndrome (specifically MDS with isolated 5q deletion)

⚙ Classic Immunophenotype
- CD41 ➕ (GPIIb/IIIa)
- CD31 ➕
- Factor VIII related antigen (vWF) ➕
- CD42b ➕ (GpIb)
- CD61 ➕ (GpIIIa)

Miscellaneous: Megakaryocytes give rise to the platelets which circulate in blood. Megakaryocytes are not present in the peripheral blood. Under normal circumstances they reside in the bone marrow and when the marrow is unable to produce them normally (e.g. primary myelofibrosis), they may be seen in other organs such as the spleen as part of extramedullary hematopoiesis. Their byproduct (platelets) are an essential part of hemostasis.

🩸 Platelets

PLATELETS

Wide variation in shape and size, usually round or elliptical

Clear or slightly blue-gray cytoplasm

On high power, can see purple or red granules (dispersed or centrally aggregated)

━━━━━━━━10µm

Rashidi H MD, Nguyen J MD et al. HematologyOutlines.com

The yellow arrows point to the relatively small-sized platelets.

🔬 Microscopic Features
- *Most are 1/5 to 1/3 the size of a normal RBC*
- They are typically round with a blue-bray cytoplasm
- Cytoplasm with purple/blue granules

⚠️ Frequency in Tissues
- Peripheral Blood: ● Many
- Bone Marrow: ✪ Scattered
- Lymph Node: ⊘ None

↔ May Resemble
- Schistocyte {p. 100}
- Stain precipitate
- Malaria Infection {p. 115}
- Babesia Infection {p. 116}

Dx Differential Diagnoses
- ↑ Increased in:
  - Iron deficiency anemia
  - Acute or chronic inflammation
  - Myeloproliferative neoplasms
  - Drug reaction
  - Exercise
- ↓ Decreased in:
  - Microangiopathic hemolytic anemias
  - Malignancy with marrow infiltration
  - Drug induced infection (e.g. sepsis leading to DIC)
  - Autoimmune (e.g. ITP)
  - Nutritional deficiencies
  - Splenic sequestration
  - Hereditary causes

⚙️ Classic Immunophenotype
- CD41 ➕
- CD42b ➕
- CD61 ➕

Miscellaneous: Platelets are the smallest cellular fragments noted on a peripheral blood smear.

🩸 Micro-Megakaryocyte

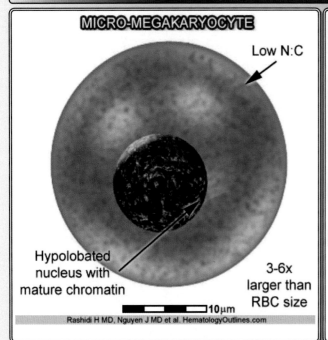

MICRO-MEGAKARYOCYTE

Low N:C

Hypolobated nucleus with mature chromatin

3-6x larger than RBC size

10µm

Rashidi H MD, Nguyen J MD et al. HematologyOutlines.com

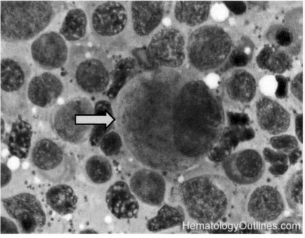

Bone marrow aspirate
The yellow arrow points to the micromegakaryocyte.

🔬 Microscopic Features
- ***3-6X larger than a mature RBC***
- Lower nuclear-to-cytoplasmic ratio because of increased cytoplasm
- Many are hypolobated (1-2 lobes) with a mature (clumped chromatin) nucleus
- Nucleoli are absent
- Cytoplasm is abundant and light blue and usually lacks granules
- Nuclear size is much smaller than normal hypolobated megakaryocytes

⚠ Frequency in Tissues
- Peripheral Blood: ⊘ None
- Bone Marrow: ⊘ None
- Lymph Node: ⊘ None

↔ May Resemble
- Megakaryocyte (normal) {p. 46}
- Osteoclast
- Histiocyte
- Monocyte {p. 40}
- Osteoblast
- Metastatic tumor cells
- Myelocyte {p. 23}

ᴅx Differential Diagnoses
Usually associated with:
- ○ MDS
- ○ Post chemotherapy etc.

⚙ Classic Immunophenotype
- CD41 ➕
- CD42b ➕
- CD61 ➕

Miscellaneous: The presence of micromegakaryocytes may be associated with a myelodysplastic syndrome (MDS).

💧 Dyslobated (Abnl Lobation) Megakaryocyte

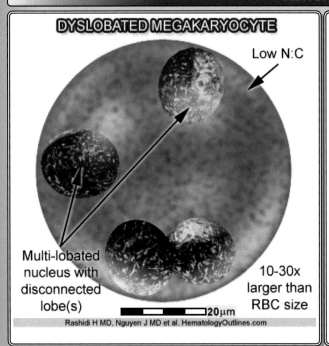

DYSLOBATED MEGAKARYOCYTE

Low N:C

Multi-lobated nucleus with disconnected lobe(s)

10-30x larger than RBC size

20µm

Rashidi H MD, Nguyen J MD et al. HematologyOutlines.com

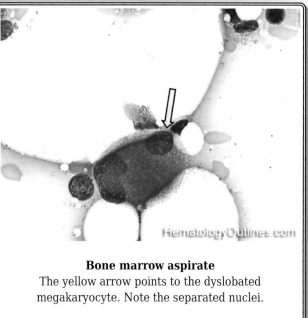

Bone marrow aspirate
The yellow arrow points to the dyslobated megakaryocyte. Note the separated nuclei.

🔬 Microscopic Features
- 10-30X larger than a mature RBC
- Lower nuclear-to-cytoplasmic ratio because of increased cytoplasm
- ***Multilobated nucleus (2-8 lobes on top of each other) with mature chromatin (clumped) but with disconnected lobe(s) (usually on the polar opposite end)***
- Nucleoli are absent
- Cytoplasm is abundant and light blue and usually lacks granules

⚠ Frequency in Tissues
- Peripheral Blood: ⊘ None
- Bone Marrow: ⊘ None
- Lymph Node: ⊘ None

↔ May Resemble
- Megakaryocyte (normal) {p. 46}
- Osteoclast
- Histiocytes and macrophages (especially multinucleated forms)
- Hodgkin Lymphoma Reed Sternberg cell (see in Glossary)
- Metastatic tumor cells

ᴰx Differential Diagnoses
Usually associated with:
- ○ MDS
- ○ Post chemotherapy etc.

⚙ Classic Immunophenotype
- CD41 ➕
- CD42 ➕
- CD61 ➕

Miscellaneous: For megakaryocytes with polar disconnected lobes, consider MDS. For megakaryocytes with staghorn-shaped nuclei, consider essential thrombocythemia (a myeloproliferative neoplasm).

🌢 Hypolobated Megakaryocytes (Increased)

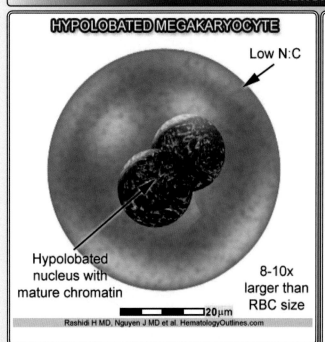

HYPOLOBATED MEGAKARYOCYTE

Low N:C

Hypolobated nucleus with mature chromatin

8-10x larger than RBC size

20μm

Rashidi H MD, Nguyen J MD et al. HematologyOutlines.com

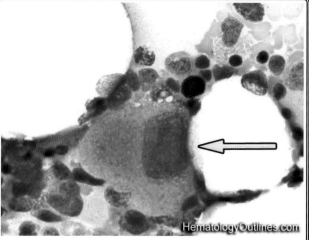

HematologyOutlines.com

Bone marrow aspirate
The yellow arrow points to the hypolobated megakaryocyte. Note the nuclear size is larger than the micromegakaryocyte.

🔬 Microscopic Features
- *8-10X larger than a mature RBC*
- Lower nuclear-to-cytoplasmic ratio because of increased cytoplasm
- Many are hypolobated (1-2 lobes) with a mature (clumped chromatin) nucleus
- Nucleoli are absent
- Cytoplasm is abundant and light blue and usually lacks granules

⚠ Frequency in Tissues
- Peripheral Blood: ⊘ None
- Bone Marrow: ○ Rare Scattered
- Lymph Node: ⊘ None

↔ May Resemble
- Megakaryocyte (normal) {p. 46}
- Osteoclast
- Histiocytes and macrophages (especially multinucleated forms)
- Osteoblast
- Hodgkin Lymphoma Reed Sternberg cell (see in Glossary)
- Metastatic tumor cells
- Myelocyte {p. 23}

Dx Differential Diagnoses
- Myelodysplastic syndrome (MDS)
- Reactive increase secondary to peripheral destruction of platelets
- Post chemotherapy toxin-induced

⚙ Classic Immunophenotype
- CD41 ⊞
- CD42b ⊞
- CD61 ⊞

Miscellaneous: Hypolobated megakaryocytes may be dysplastic and associated with a myelodysplastic syndrome (MDS) or newly forming megakaryocytes that are the result of a peripheral destruction of platelets (e.g. ITP).

💧 Staghorn-shaped Megakaryocyte

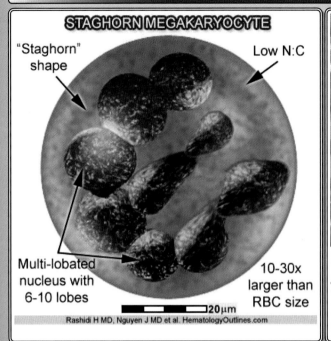

STAGHORN MEGAKARYOCYTE

"Staghorn" shape

Low N:C

Multi-lobated nucleus with 6-10 lobes

10-30x larger than RBC size

20μm

Rashidi H MD, Nguyen J MD et al. HematologyOutlines.com

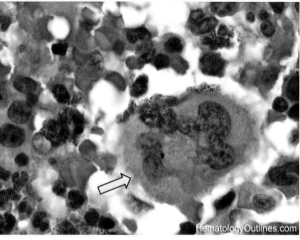

Bone marrow aspirate

The yellow arrow points to the staghorn megakaryocyte.

🔬 Microscopic Features

- 10-30X larger than a mature RBC
- Lower nuclear-to-cytoplasmic ratio because of increased cytoplasm
- *Multilobated nucleus (6-10 lobes with a staghorn configuration)*
- Nucleoli are absent
- Cytoplasm is abundant and light blue which usually lacks granules

⚠️ Frequency in Tissues

- Peripheral Blood: ⊘ None
- Bone Marrow: ⊘ None
- Lymph Node: ⊘ None

↔ May Resemble

- Megakaryocyte (normal) {p. 46}
- Osteoclast
- Histiocytes and macrophages (especially multinucleated forms)
- Hodgkin Lymphoma Reed Sternberg cell (see in Glossary)
- Metastatic tumor cells

Dx Differential Diagnoses

- Myeloproliferative neoplasm (specifically essential thrombocythemia (ET))
- Post chemotherapy MDS (rarely)

⚙ Classic Immunophenotype

- CD41 ⊞
- CD42 ⊞
- CD61 ⊞

Miscellaneous: For megakaryocytes with polar disconnected lobes, consider MDS. For megakaryocytes with staghorn-shaped nuclei, consider essential thrombocythemia (a myeloproliferative neoplasm).

⬥ Megakaryoblast (Increased)

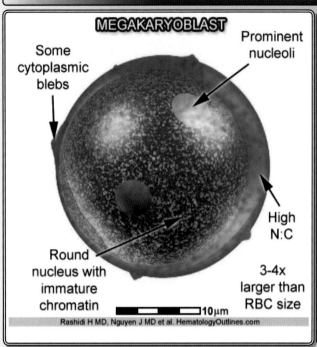

MEGAKARYOBLAST

Some cytoplasmic blebs

Prominent nucleoli

Round nucleus with immature chromatin

High N:C

3-4x larger than RBC size

10μm

Rashidi H MD, Nguyen J MD et al. HematologyOutlines.com

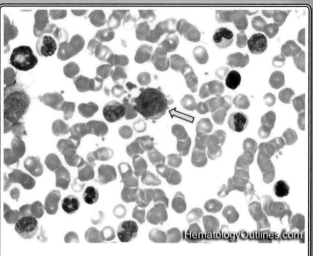

The yellow arrow points to the megakaryoblast. Note the nucleolus and the cytoplasmic blebs.

🔬 Microscopic Features

- 3-4X larger than a mature RBC
- **High nuclear-to-cytoplasmic ratio**
- Round nucleus with immature chromatin (not clumped)
- Prominent nucleoli
- Cytoplasm is pale blue with occasional cytoplasmic blebs (want-to-be platelets)

⚠ Frequency in Tissues

- Peripheral Blood: ⊘ None
- Bone Marrow: ○ Rare (<1%)
- Lymph Node: ⊘ None

↔ May Resemble

- Myeloblast {p. 21}
- Pronormoblast {p. 9}
- Lymphoblast {p. 65}
- Immature B-cell (hematogone) {p. 62}
- Monoblast {p. 38}
- Reactive Lymphocyte {p. 137}

ᴰx Differential Diagnoses

- Acute megakaryoblastic leukemia (AML-M7)
- Transient myelopoeisis (usually associated with some newborns with Down syndrome)

⚙ Classic Immunophenotype

- CD41 ➕
- CD42b ➖
- CD61 ➕

Miscellaneous: Transient myelopoiesis also shows increased megakaryoblasts in the peripheral blood and/or bone marrow of a newborn Down syndrome patient and may mimic an AML-M7 (acute megakaryoblastic leukemia).

Bone Marrow: Lymphoid Overview Mindmap

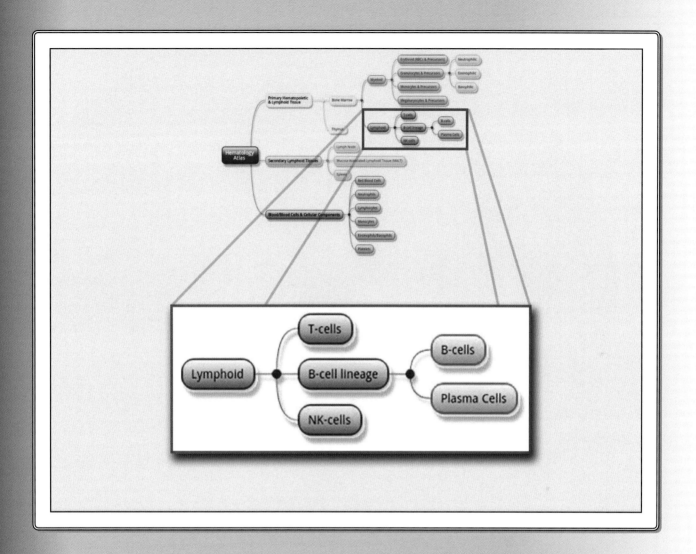

T-cell Maturation Diagram

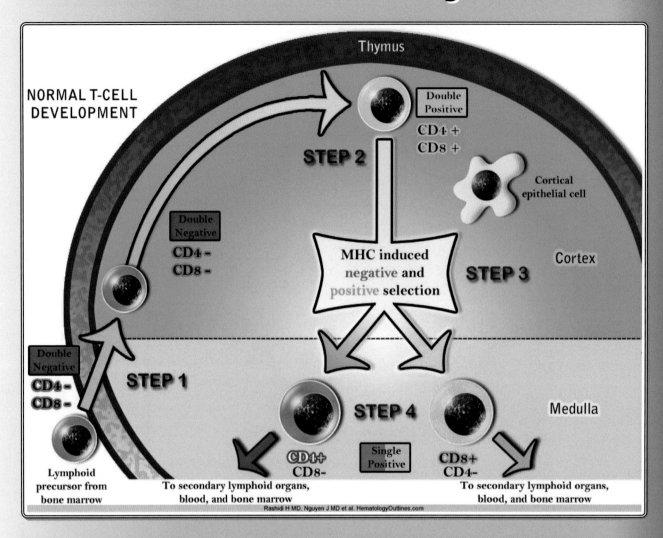

Rashidi H MD, Nguyen J MD et al. HematologyOutlines.com

T-cells start in the bone marrow as T-cell precursors, and then leave the bone marrow to enter the thymus to undergo maturation. Upon maturation they then leave the thymus to enter circulation (blood) and other tissues (e.g. secondary lymphoid tissues). The above diagram shows the immature Double Negative (CD4-/CD8-) T-cell entering the thymus at the corticomedullary junction to eventually progess in the cortex to become Double Positive (CD4+/CD8+) T-cells that undergo further maturation to eventually enter the medullary portion of the thymus as CD4+/CD8- or CD4-/CD8+ (Single Positive) T-cells.

In summary: The T-cells start as CD4-/CD8-(Double Negative), then become CD4+/CD8+ (Double Positive), and following a MHC induced positive and negative selection process, they eventually become mature CD4+/CD8- or CD4-/CD8+ (Single Positive) T-cells which will enter blood and various tissues. Note that in contrast to the B-cells which start their early maturation in the bone marrow, T-cells start their maturation process in the thymus. Mnemonic is "B" for B-cells and Bone marrow and "T" for T-cells and thymus. Within one T-cell maturation scheme, the T-cell receptor (TCR) gene rearrangement occurs in a predictable ordered fashion with the γ (gamma) and δ (delta) genes rearranging before the α (alpha) and β (beta) genes in the double negative stage of the T-cells. The γ/δ rearrangements that do not give rise to functional γ/δ TCR proteins will then undergo α and β gene rearrangement to ultimately give rise to a functional α/β type TCR protein which comprises the vast majority of the TCR proteins.

⬥ Immature T-cell precursor

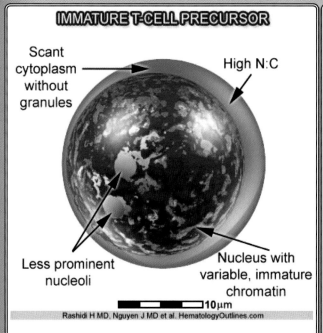

IMMATURE T-CELL PRECURSOR

Scant cytoplasm without granules

High N:C

Less prominent nucleoli

Nucleus with variable, immature chromatin

10μm

Rashidi H MD, Nguyen J MD et al. HematologyOutlines.com

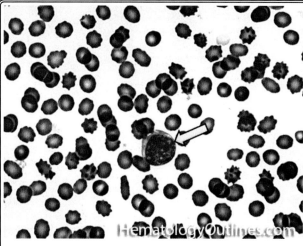

The yellow arrow points to the immature T-cell.

🔬 Microscopic Features
- 3-4X larger than a mature RBC
- *High nuclear-to-cytoplasmic ratio*
- Round nucleus with immature chromatin (not clumped)
- Prominent nucleoli
- Cytoplasm is scant, light blue and lacks granules

⚠ Frequency in Tissues
- Peripheral Blood: ⊘ None
- Bone Marrow: ○ Rare (~1%)
- Lymph Node: ⊘ None

↔ May Resemble
- Myeloblast {p. 21}
- Pronormoblast {p. 9}
- Immature B-cell (hematogone) {p. 62}
- Monoblast {p. 38}
- Prolymphocyte
- Reactive Lymphocyte {p. 137}

℞x Differential Diagnoses
- T-Lymphoblastic leukemia (T-ALL)
- Rarely some non-neoplastic conditions

⚙ Classic Immunophenotype
- CD1a ⊞/⊖
- Tdt ⊞/⊖
- CD2 ⊞/⊖
- CD3 (cytoplasmic) ⊞/⊖
- CD4 ⊞/⊖ and CD8 ⊞/⊖
- CD5 ⊞/⊖
- CD7 ⊞

Miscellaneous: Very immature cells cannot be reliably distinguished from each other based on morphology alone. The exception are blasts with Auer rod(s) which are unique to abnormal myeloblasts and abnormal promyelocytes as noted in acute promyelocytic leukemia (APL).

◊ Mature T-cells

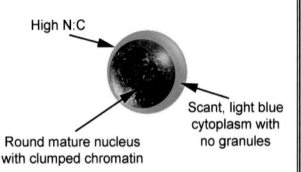

MATURE T-CELL

Slightly larger than mature RBC

High N:C

Round mature nucleus with clumped chromatin

Scant, light blue cytoplasm with no granules

⊨▬▬▬▬▬□▬▬▬▬▬10µm

Rashidi H MD, Nguyen J MD et al. HematologyOutlines.com

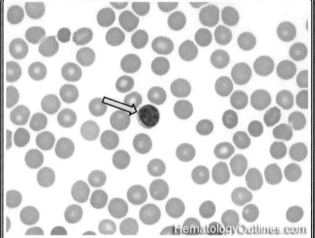

HematologyOutlines.com

The yellow arrow points to the mature lymphocyte. Note the nuclear size which is slightly larger than the size of a red blood cell.

🔬 Microscopic Features
- *Slightly (~1.5X) larger than a mature RBC*
- High nuclear-to-cytoplasmic ratio but with round mature nucleus (clumped chromatin)
- Nucleoli are absent
- Cytoplasm is scant, light blue and lacks granules

⚠ Frequency in Tissues
- Peripheral Blood: ● 2nd most common nucleated cell (WBC) in blood and most common lymphocyte in blood
- Bone Marrow: ✪ Scattered (<10%)
- Lymph Node: ✪ Mainly scattered in interfollicular areas of lymphoid tissue

↔ May Resemble
- Mature B-cells (can't distinguish T-cell and B-cell based on morphology)
- Orthochromic Normoblast {p. 12}
- Plasma Cell (mature) {p. 67}
- Reactive Lymphocyte {p. 137}
- Monocyte {p. 40}

Dx Differential Diagnoses
- Infection
- Neoplastic (mature T-cell lymphoma or leukemia)
- Drug-induced
- Autoimmune disorders
- Idiopathic

⚙ Classic Immunophenotype
- CD2 ➕
- CD3 ➕
- CD4 ➕ or CD8 ➕
- CD5 ➕
- CD7 ➕
- TCR ➕ (usually α/β subtype), <5% γ/δ ➕
- TdT ➖
- CD34 ➖

Miscellaneous: Morphologically you cannot distinguish mature T-cells from mature B-cells. Within the peripheral blood, there are more CD4+ T-cells than CD8+ T-cells (CD4:CD8 ratio is ~2-3:1). The majority of the mature T-cells express the α/β TCR (only a small minority express the γ/δ TCR).

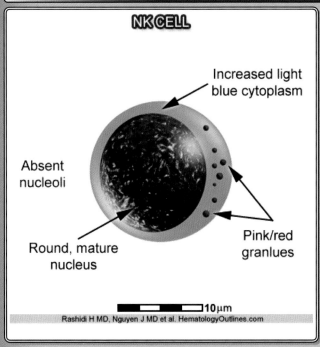

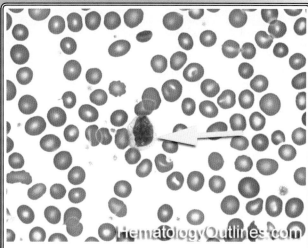

The yellow arrow points to the slightly large and irregular lymphocyte which usually contains granules.

🔬 Microscopic Features
- *Slightly larger than a mature RBC*
- High nuclear-to-cytoplasmic ratio but with a round mature nucleus (clumped chromatin)
- Nucleoli are absent
- Cytoplasm may have some granules

⚠ Frequency in Tissues
- Peripheral Blood: ○ Rare (lymphocytes in general are the 2nd most common WBCs in blood. Majority are T-cells, followed by scattered B-cells and rare scattered NK-cells)
- Bone Marrow: ○ Rare
- Lymph Node: ○ Rare

↔ May Resemble
- Mature T-LGL cell (cannot distinguish it from mature T-cell or B-cells based on morphology)
- Reactive Lymphocyte {p. 137}
- Monocyte {p. 40}

Dx Differential Diagnoses
- Infection
- Neoplastic (NK cell leukemia and lymphoma)

⚙ Classic Immunophenotype
- Surface CD3 ⊖ (in contrast to T-cells which are ⊕)
- CD2 ⊕ (similar to T-cells)
- CD5 ⊖ (in contrast to T-cells which are ⊕)
- CD7 ⊕ (similar to T-cells)
- CD8 subset **dim** ⊕ / ⊖
- TCR ⊖ (in contrast to T-cells which are ⊕)
- Cytoplasmic CD3-ε (epsilon) chain ⊕
- CD56 ⊕

Miscellaneous: Morphologically you cannot distinguish NK cells from T-cells or LGLs.

🜄 T-Lymphoblasts (Increased)

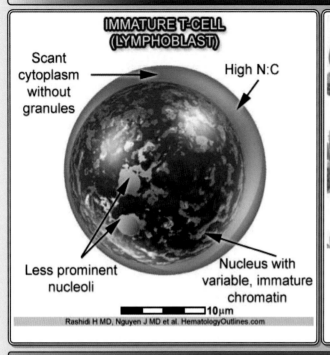

IMMATURE T-CELL (LYMPHOBLAST)

Scant cytoplasm without granules

High N:C

Less prominent nucleoli

Nucleus with variable, immature chromatin

10μm

Rashidi H MD, Nguyen J MD et al. HematologyOutlines.com

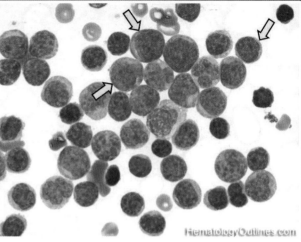

The yellow arrows depict the increase in immature cells.

🔬 Microscopic Features
- 3-4X larger than a mature RBC
- **High nuclear-to-cytoplasmic ratio**
- Round nucleus with immature chromatin (not clumped)
- Prominent nucleoli
- Cytoplasm is scant, light blue and lacks granules

⚠ Frequency in Tissues
- Peripheral Blood: ⊘ None
- Bone Marrow: ○ Rare (~1%)
- Lymph Node: ⊘ None

↔ May Resemble
- Myeloblast {p. 21}
- Pronormoblast {p. 9}
- Immature B-cell (hematogone) {p. 62}
- Monoblast {p. 38}
- Prolymphocyte
- Reactive Lymphocyte {p. 137}

℞x Differential Diagnoses
- T-Lymphoblastic leukemia (T-ALL)
- Rarely some non-neoplastic conditions

⚙ Classic Immunophenotype
- CD2 ➕ / ➖
- CD3 ➕ / ➖
- CD5 ➕ / ➖
- CD7 ➕
- CD34 ➕ / ➖ and TdT ➕ / ➖
- The immunotype depends on the subtype of T-lymphoblast (CD4 ➕ / CD8 ➕ or CD4 ➖ / CD8 ➖ are most common)

Miscellaneous: Blast cells cannot be reliably distinguished from each other based on morphology alone. The exception are blasts with Auer rod(s) which are unique to abnormal myeloblasts and abnormal promyelocytes as noted in some AMLs and APL.

📓 **Note**: Abnormal lymphoblasts can show immunophenotypic aberrancies (e.g. loss of T-cell antigens such as CD7, CD5 and CD2 or the gain of myeloid markers such as CD13, etc.).

◊ Large Granular Lymphocyte (LGL)

ABNORMAL

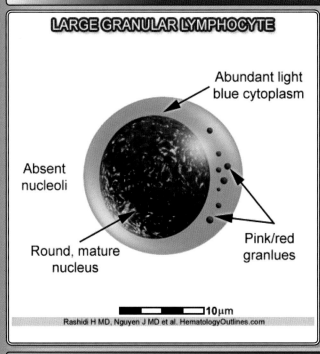

LARGE GRANULAR LYMPHOCYTE

Abundant light blue cytoplasm

Absent nucleoli

Round, mature nucleus

Pink/red granlues

⊢10μm

Rashidi H MD, Nguyen J MD et al. HematologyOutlines.com

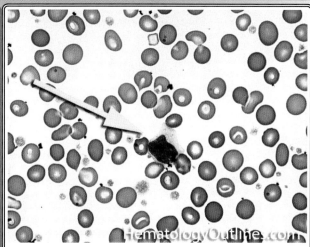

The yellow arrow points to the large granular lymphocyte. Note the large reddish granules in the cytoplasm.

🔬 Microscopic Features
- 2-4X larger than a mature RBC
- Low nuclear-to-cytoplasmic ratio because of the increased cytoplasm
- Round-to-convoluted nuclear border with mature chromatin (clumped chromatin)
- Nucleoli are absent
- Cytoplasm is abundant and light blue
- *Pink/red granules seen within the cytoplasm (hence the term "granular")*

⚠ Frequency in Tissues
- Peripheral Blood: ○ Rare to ⊘ None
- Bone Marrow: ⊘ None
- Lymph Node: ⊘ None

↔ May Resemble
- Reactive Lymphocyte {p. 137}
- NK Cells {p. 57}
- Monocyte {p. 40}
- Promyelocyte {p. 22}

Dx Differential Diagnoses
- Infection/inflammatory conditions
- Neoplastic (LGL leukemia)

⚙ Classic Immunophenotype
- CD2 ➕
- CD3 ➕
- CD4 ➖
- CD8 ➕
- CD5 ➕
- CD7 ➕
- CD16 ➕
- CD56 ➕ / ➖
- CD57 ➕

Miscellaneous: Must rule out reactive conditions (e.g. infection, etc.) before considering LGL leukemia as a diagnosis.

♦ Increased Mature T-cells

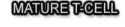
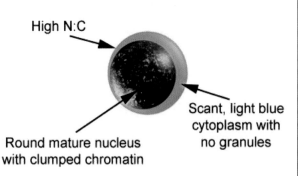

MATURE T-CELL

Slightly larger than mature RBC

High N:C

Round mature nucleus with clumped chromatin

Scant, light blue cytoplasm with no granules

⊏━━━━━⊐10µm

Rashidi H MD, Nguyen J MD et al. HematologyOutlines.com

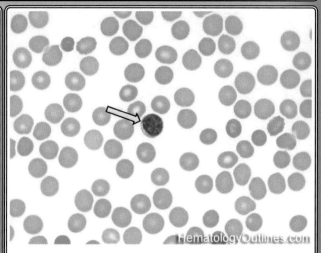

The yellow arrow points to the mature lymphocyte.

🔬 Microscopic Features
- *Slightly (~1.5X) larger than a mature RBC (activated T-cells may be 2-3X the size of a normal RBC)*
- High nuclear-to-cytoplasmic ratio but with round mature nucleus (clumped chromatin)
- Nucleoli are absent
- Cytoplasm is scant, light blue and lacks granules

⚠ Frequency in Tissues
- Peripheral Blood: ● 2nd most common nucleated cell (WBC) in blood and most common lymphocyte in blood
- Bone Marrow: ❀ Scattered (<10%)
- Lymph Node: ❀ Mainly scattered in interfollicular areas of lymphoid tissue

↔ May Resemble
- Mature B-cells (can't distinguish T-cell and B-cell based on morphology)
- Orthochromic Normoblast {p. 12}
- Plasma Cell (mature) {p. 67}
- Reactive Lymphocyte {p. 137}
- Monocyte {p. 40}

ᴅₓ Differential Diagnoses
- Infection
- Neoplastic (mature T-cell lymphoma or leukemia)
- Drug-induced
- Autoimmune disorders
- Idiopathic

⚙ Classic Immunophenotype
- CD2 ➕
- CD3 ➕
- CD4 ➕ or CD8 ➕
- CD5 ➕
- CD7 ➕
- TCR ➕
- TdT ➖
- CD34 ➖

Miscellaneous: Morphologically you cannot distinguish mature T-cells from mature B-cells. Within the peripheral blood, there are more CD4+ T-cells than CD8+ T-cells (CD4:CD8 ratio is ~2-3:1). The majority of the mature T-cells express the α/β TCR (only a small minority express the γ/δ TCR).

B-cell Maturation Diagram

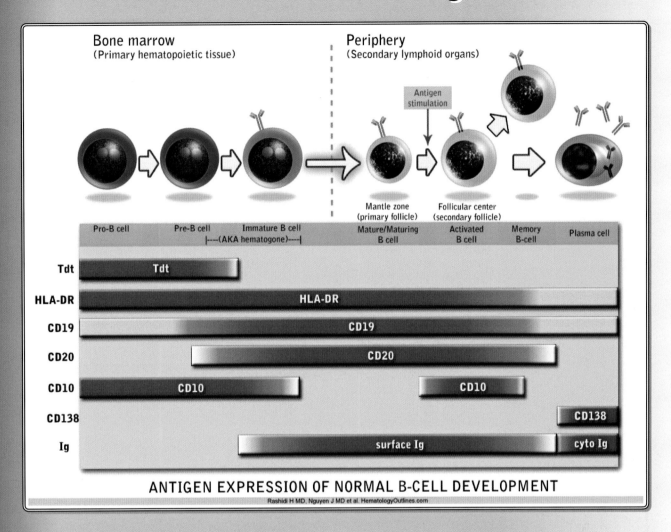

Bone marrow
(Primary hematopoietic tissue)

Periphery
(Secondary lymphoid organs)

Antigen stimulation

Mantle zone (primary follicle)

Follicular center (secondary follicle)

	Pro-B cell	Pre-B cell	Immature B cell |----(AKA hematogone)----|	Mature/Maturing B cell	Activated B cell	Memory B-cell	Plasma cell
Tdt	Tdt						
HLA-DR	HLA-DR						
CD19	CD19						
CD20		CD20					
CD10	CD10			CD10			
CD138							CD138
Ig		surface Ig					cyto Ig

ANTIGEN EXPRESSION OF NORMAL B-CELL DEVELOPMENT

Rashidi H MD, Nguyen J MD et al. HematologyOutlines.com

B-cell maturation starts with B-cell precursors in the bone marrow. These precursors progress to becoming hematogones (various stages of immature B-cells in the bone marrow) and then become early maturing B-cells in the bone marrow. These early maturing B-cells then leave the bone marrow and end up in secondary lymphoid tissues (e.g. Lymph nodes, MALT or Spleen) where they finish their maturation process upon antigen stimulation (During pre-antigen stimulation, these B-cells are predominantly in primary follicles and upon antigen stimulation they enter the germinal center of secondary follicles where somatic hypermutation and class switching occurs that eventually give rise to memory B-cells and plasma cells). TdT is confined to the very early B-cells in bone marrow (early hematogones) only. CD20 is not expressed in early hematogones or plasma cells but rather relatively confined to maturing/mature B-cells. CD10 is expressed in two distinct stages: within hematogones and then in germinal centers. CD138 is relatively confined to plasma cells, although it may also be expressed in non-hematopoietic cell lines such as epithelial cells.

As opposed to B-cells that have surface bound immunoglobulins (Ig), the Ig of plasma cells are cytoplasmic because they are made to be secreted. Additionally, as opposed to both B-cells and T-cells which circulate in the peripheral blood, plasma cells are usually absent in blood. Note: All B-cells express some level of CD19 and as antigen presenting cells they would be expected to also express MHC class II molecules which explains the expression of HLA-DR (a MHC class II) on all B-cells (from early B-cells to plasma cells).

◊ Immature B-cell (Early Hematogone)

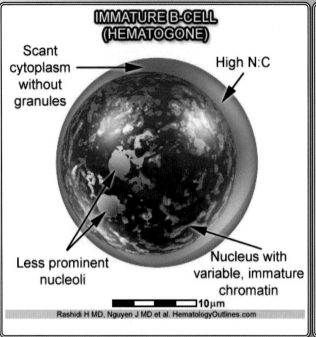

IMMATURE B-CELL (HEMATOGONE)

Scant cytoplasm without granules

High N:C

Less prominent nucleoli

Nucleus with variable, immature chromatin

10μm

Rashidi H MD, Nguyen J MD et al. HematologyOutlines.com

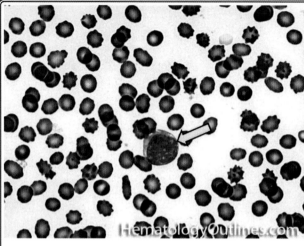

Bone marrow aspirate
The yellow arrow points to the immature lymphocyte with visible nucleoli.

🔬 Microscopic Features
- 3-4X larger than a mature RBC
- *High nuclear-to-cytoplasmic ratio*
- Round nucleus with immature chromatin (not clumped)
- Prominent nucleoli
- Cytoplasm is scant, light blue and lacks granules

⚠ Frequency in Tissues
- Peripheral Blood: ⊘ None
- Bone Marrow: 1%
- Lymph Node: ⊘ None

↔ May Resemble
- Myeloblast {p. 21}
- Pronormoblast {p. 9}
- Immature T-cell {p. 55}
- Monoblast {p. 38}
- Reactive Lymphocyte {p. 137}

℞x Differential Diagnoses
- May be increased in newborns (not to be confused with acute leukemia)
- May be seen in recovering bone marrow (e.g. post-treatment)
- Acute leukemia

⚙ Classic Immunophenotype
- CD19 ➕
- CD10 ➕
- CD20 ➖ , PAX5 ➕
- CD34 ➕
- CD38 ➕➕
- TdT ➕
- Kappa ➖ and Lambda ➖
- CD45 **very dim** ➕

Miscellaneous: Very immature cells cannot be reliably distinguished from each other based on morphology alone. The exception are blasts with Auer rod(s) which are unique to abnormal myeloblasts and abnormal promyelocytes as noted in some AMLs and APL. These are immature B-cells that are usually morphologically indistinguishable from lymphoblasts. Hematogones are a immunophenotypically diverse group of immature B-cells (earlier forms have less mature markers such as CD34 and TdT while the more mature forms lack CD34 and TdT and partially express CD20).

🔵 Immature B-cell (Later Hematogone)

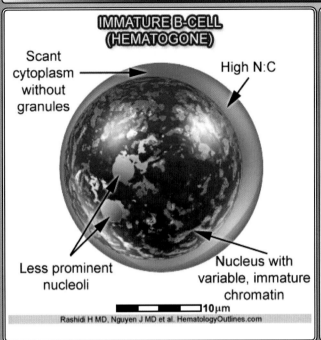

IMMATURE B-CELL (HEMATOGONE)

Scant cytoplasm without granules

High N:C

Less prominent nucleoli

Nucleus with variable, immature chromatin

10μm

Rashidi H MD, Nguyen J MD et al. HematologyOutlines.com

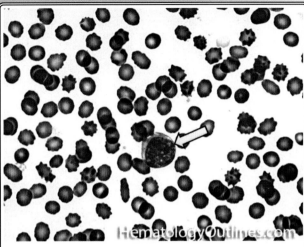

Bone marrow aspirate
The yellow arrow points to the immature lymphocyte.
Note the nucleoli.

🔬 Microscopic Features
- *2-4X larger than a mature RBC (variable size given their variable stage of maturation)*
- High nuclear-to-cytoplasmic ratio
- Round nucleus with immature chromatin (not clumped)
- Nucleoli are present (especially on less mature stages) but less prominent than blasts
- Cytoplasm is scant, light blue and lacks granules
- *Usually it is morphologically indistinguishable from a lymphoblast*

⚠️ Frequency in Tissues
- Peripheral Blood: ⊘ None
- Bone Marrow: ✦ Scattered
- Lymph Node: ⊘ None

↔️ May Resemble
- Myeloblast {p. 21}
- Pronormoblast {p. 9}
- Immature B-cell (hematogone) {p. 62}
- Monoblast {p. 38}
- Reactive Lymphocyte {p. 137}

ᴰˣ Differential Diagnoses
- May be increased in newborns (not to be confused with acute leukemia)
- May be seen in recovering bone marrow (e.g. post-treatment)
- Acute leukemia

⚙️ Classic Immunophenotype
- CD19 ⊞
- CD10 ⊞
- CD20 ⊞ / ⊖ , PAX5 ⊞
- CD38 ⊞ ⊞
- CD45 **dim** ⊞
- CD34 ⊖
- TdT ⊖
- Kappa ⊖ and Lambda ⊖

Miscellaneous: These are immature B-cells that are usually morphologically indistinguishable from lymphoblasts. Hematogones are a immunophenotypically diverse group of immature B-cells (earlier forms have less mature markers such as CD34 and TdT while the more mature forms lack CD34 and TdT and partially express CD20).

◊ Mature B-cells

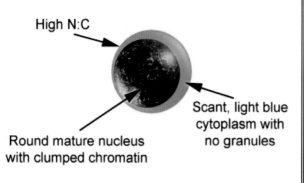

MATURE B-CELL

Slightly larger than
mature RBC

High N:C

Round mature nucleus
with clumped chromatin

Scant, light blue
cytoplasm with
no granules

10µm

Rashidi H MD, Nguyen J MD et al. HematologyOutlines.com

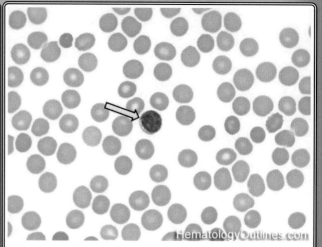

The yellow arrow points to the mature small
lymphocyte.

🔬 Microscopic Features
- *Slightly (1.5X) larger than a mature RBC*
- High nuclear-to-cytoplasmic ratio but with round mature nucleus (clumped chromatin)
- Nucleoli are absent
- Cytoplasm is scant, light blue and lacks granules

⚠ Frequency in Tissues
- Peripheral Blood: 2nd most common lymphocyte after T-cells
- Bone Marrow: ○ Rare
- Lymph Node: ✷ Mainly distributed in follicular areas (germinal centers and mantle zones)

↔ May Resemble
- Mature T-cells (cannot distinguish T-cell and B-cell based on morphology)
- Reactive Lymphocyte {p. 137}
- Monocyte {p. 40}

℞ₓ Differential Diagnoses
- Infection
- Neoplastic (mature B-cell lymphoma or leukemia such as CLL)

⚙ Classic Immunophenotype
- CD19 ⊕
- CD20 ⊕ , PAX5 ⊕
- CD22 ⊕
- TdT ⊖
- CD34 ⊖
- Kappa and Lambda polytypic

Miscellaneous: Morphologically, one cannot distinguish mature T-cells from mature B-cells.

🩸 Increased B-Lymphoblasts

ABNORMAL

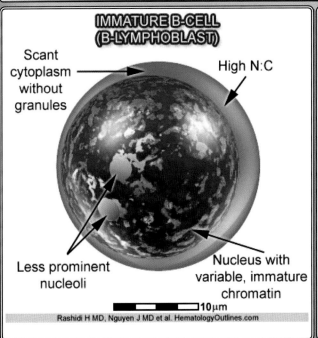

IMMATURE B-CELL
(B-LYMPHOBLAST)

Scant cytoplasm without granules

High N:C

Less prominent nucleoli

Nucleus with variable, immature chromatin

⊢——⊣10µm

Rashidi H MD, Nguyen J MD et al. HematologyOutlines.com

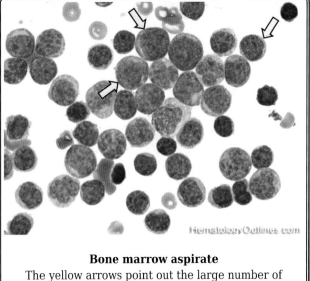

Bone marrow aspirate
The yellow arrows point out the large number of lymphoblasts.

🔬 Microscopic Features
- 3-4X larger than a mature RBC
- *High nuclear-to-cytoplasmic ratio*
- Round nucleus with immature chromatin (not clumped)
- Prominent nucleoli
- Cytoplasm is scant, light blue and lacks granules

⚠ Frequency in Tissues
- Peripheral Blood: ⊘ None
- Bone Marrow: ⊘ None
- Lymph Node: ⊘ None

↔ May Resemble
- Myeloblast {p. 21}
- Pronormoblast {p. 9}
- Immature B-cell (hematogone) {p. 62}
- Monoblast {p. 38}
- Prolymphocyte
- Reactive Lymphocyte {p. 137}

Dx Differential Diagnoses
- B-cell acute lymphoblastic leukemia/lymphoma (B-ALL)
- CML: lymphoblastic blast crisis (usually myeloblasts but can sometimes be lymphoblasts)

⚙ Classic Immunophenotype
- CD19 ⊞
- CD10 ⊞
- CD20 ⊟ / ⊞
- CD34 ⊞
- CD38 ⊞ / ⊟
- Kappa ⊟ and Lambda ⊟
- TdT ⊞

Miscellaneous: Blasts cannot be reliably distinguished from each other based on morphology alone. The exception are blasts with Auer rod(s) which are unique to abnormal myeloblasts and abnormal promyelocytes as noted in some AMLs and APL.

Note: Abnormal B-lymphoblasts can show immunophenotypic abberancies (e.g. the gain of myeloid markers).

🩸 Increased Mature Appearing B-cells

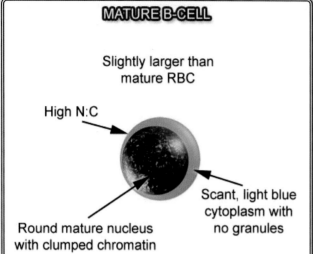

MATURE B-CELL

Slightly larger than mature RBC

High N:C

Round mature nucleus with clumped chromatin

Scant, light blue cytoplasm with no granules

10μm

Rashidi H MD, Nguyen J MD et al. HematologyOutlines.com

Note that the only white blood cells seen in this field of view are small mature lymphocytes.

🔬 Microscopic Features
- *Slightly (1.5X) larger than a mature RBC*
- High nuclear-to-cytoplasmic ratio but with round mature nucleus (clumped chromatin)
- Nucleoli are absent
- Cytoplasm is scant, light blue and lacks granules

⚠ Frequency in Tissues
- Peripheral Blood: ⊘ None (abnormal lymphocytes are rarely present)
- Bone Marrow: ⊘ None (abnormal lymphocytes are rarely present)
- Lymph Node: ⊘ None (abnormal lymphocytes are rarely present)

↔ May Resemble
- Mature T-cells (cannot distinguish T-cell and B-cell based on morphology)
- Reactive Lymphocyte {p. 137}
- Monocyte {p. 40}

Dx Differential Diagnoses
- Infection
- Neoplastic (mature B-cell lymphoma or leukemia such as but not limited to CLL or follicular lymphoma)

⚙ Classic Immunophenotype
- CD19 ➕
- CD20 ➕
- CD22 ➕
- TdT ➖
- CD34 ➖

Miscellaneous: Morphologically, one cannot distinguish mature T-cells from mature B-cells.

Note: Neoplastic mature B-cells are clonal processes which can be distinguished by their light chain restriction (kappa restricted or lambda restricted) along with their characteristic immunophenotype (e.g. CD5 and CD23 expression in CLL, etc.).

NORMAL

PLASMA CELL

Round, eccentric nucleus with coarse chromatin (may have "clock face")

Abundant basophilic cytoplasm

Prominent perinuclear hof (clearing)

10µm

Rashidi H MD, Nguyen J MD et al. HematologyOutlines.com

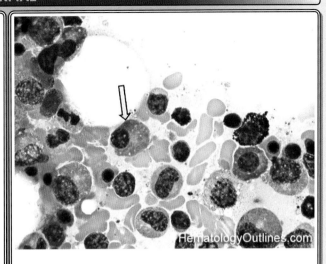

Bone marrow aspirate
The yellow arrow points to a mature plasma cell.

🔬 Microscopic Features
- 2-3X larger than a mature RBC
- *Round eccentricly placed nucleus with coarse chromatin (nucleus may show a clock-faced chromatin pattern)*
- Abundant basophilic (blue) cytoplasm with prominent perinuclear hof (clearing)
- Nucleoli are absent

⚠ Frequency in Tissues
- Peripheral Blood: ⊘ None
- Bone Marrow: ✷ Scattered
- Lymph Node: ✷ Scattered

↔ May Resemble
- Plasmablast {p. 69}
- Polychromatophilic Normoblast {p. 11}
- Osteoblast
- Mature Lymphocyte {p. 64}
- Reactive Lymphocyte {p. 137}

ᴰₓ Differential Diagnoses
- Chronic infection
- Malignancies (e.g. plasma cell myeloma, lymphoma, etc.)
- Autoimmune disorder
- Drug reaction

⚙ Classic Immunophenotype
- CD138 ➕
- CD38 bright ➕
- CD79a ➕
- MUM1 ➕
- CD19 ➕
- CD20 ➖
- CD56 ➖
- Polytypic with normal ratio of cytoplasmic kappa and lambda light chains

Miscellaneous: Plasma cells are normally seen scattered in bone marrow and lymphoid tissue. They are not seen in normal peripheral blood. The plasma cells in a normal bone marrow are polytypic (not clonal) and do not form sheets or clusters. Polytypic means a mixture of kappa and lambda light chains.

🔹 Plasma Cell Myeloma (Multiple Myeloma)

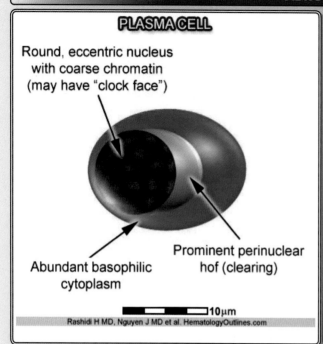

PLASMA CELL

Round, eccentric nucleus with coarse chromatin (may have "clock face")

Abundant basophilic cytoplasm

Prominent perinuclear hof (clearing)

10µm

Rashidi H MD, Nguyen J MD et al. HematologyOutlines.com

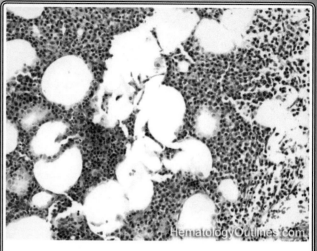

Bone marrow biopsy
Notice how the bone marrow is diffusely involved by sheets of plasma cells.

🔬 Microscopic Features
- *Usually presents as sheets or clusters of plasma cells in the bone marrow*
- Each plasma cell is 2-3X larger than a mature RBC
- Round eccentrically placed nucleus with coarse chromatin (may show a clock-faced chromatin pattern)
- Abundant basophilic (blue) cytoplasm with prominent perinuclear hof (clearing)
- Nucleoli are usually absent (some may have immature features such as prominent nucleoli)
- Other abnormal features may include nuclear pseudoinclusions known as "Dutcher Bodies"

⚠ Frequency in Tissues
- Peripheral Blood: ⊘ None
- Bone Marrow: ⊘ None
- Lymph Node: ⊘ None

↔ May Resemble
- Plasmablast {p. 69}
- Polychromatophilic Normoblast {p. 11}
- Osteoblast
- Mature Lymphocyte {p. 64}
- Reactive Lymphocyte {p. 137}

🅓x Differential Diagnoses
- MGUS
- Lymphoplasmacytic lymphoma (LPL)
- Marginal zone lymphoma
- Plasmablastic lymphoma
- Chronic infection, autoimmune disorder, drug reaction

⚙ Classic Immunophenotype
- CD138 ➕ and CD38 bright ➕ ➕
- CD19 ➖ and CD20 ➖
- CD56 ➕ (common)
- Cytoplasmic light chain restricted (kappa or lambda)

Miscellaneous: The plasma cells in plasma cell myeloma are monotypic (clonal) and typically involve the bone marrow as sheets or clusters of plasma cells. Monotypic refers to being either kappa or lambda light chain restricted (as opposed to normal polytypic plasma cells which have a mix of kappa and lambda expression). In **symptomatic plasma cell myeloma**, patients present with one or more of the "CRAB" findings: "C" for hyperCalcemia, "R" for Renal insufficiency (secondary), "A" for Anemia associated with the disease, and "B" for Bone Lesions (lytic). The new recommendations also include free light chain study since ratios of > 100:1 may change the management of some myeloma patients. Also having >60% plasma cells by CD138 IHC may change therapy as well.

⬥ Plasmablast (Immature plasma cell)

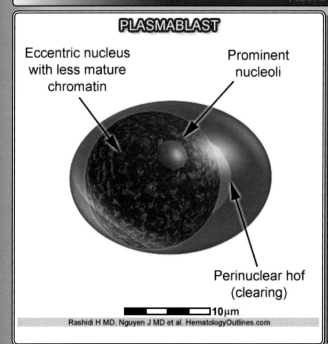

PLASMABLAST

Eccentric nucleus with less mature chromatin

Prominent nucleoli

Perinuclear hof (clearing)

⊢■□■□■10µm

Rashidi H MD, Nguyen J MD et al. HematologyOutlines.com

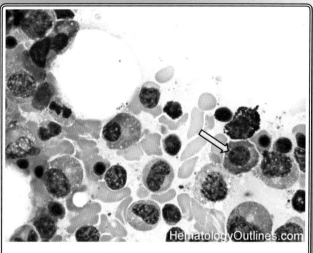

Bone marrow aspirate
The yellow arrow points to the immature plasma cell with a prominent nucleolus.

🔬 Microscopic Features
- 3-4X larger than a mature RBC
- Round eccentricly placed nucleus with less mature chromatin
- Moderate amount of basophilic (blue) cytoplasm with prominent perinuclear hof (clearing)
- ***Nucleoli are prominent***

⚠ Frequency in Tissues
- Peripheral Blood: ⊘ None
- Bone Marrow: ⊘ None
- Lymph Node: ⊘ None

↔ May Resemble
- Polychromatophilic Normoblast {p. 11}
- Plasma Cell (mature) {p. 67}
- Myeloblast {p. 21}
- Osteoblast
- Pronormoblast {p. 9}
- Monoblast {p. 38}
- Reactive Lymphocyte {p. 137}

ᴰx Differential Diagnoses
- Plasma cell myeloma (plasmablastic form)
- Plasmablastic lymphoma
- Plasma cell leukemia
- Rare forms can also be seen in reactive conditions

⚙ Classic Immunophenotype
- CD138 ⊞ and CD38 bright ⊞ ⊞
- CD19 ⊖ and CD20 ⊖
- CD56 ⊖ (more common)
- Cytoplasmic light chain restricted (kappa or lambda, in neoplastic plasma cells)

Miscellaneous: Plasmablasts are rarely found in normal bone marrow.

Primary Lymphoid Tissue: Thymus Overview Mindmap

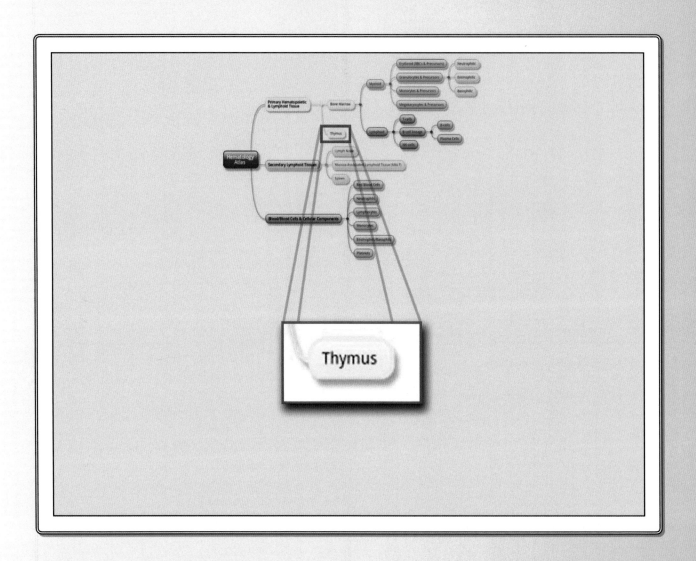

T-cell Maturation in Thymus Diagram

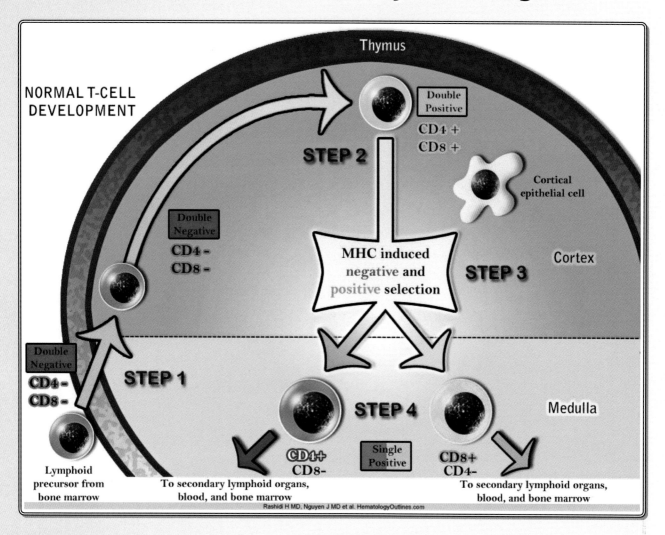

Rashidi H MD, Nguyen J MD et al. HematologyOutlines.com

T-cells start in the bone marrow as T-cell precursors, and then leave the bone marrow to enter the thymus to undergo maturation. Upon maturation they then leave the thymus to enter circulation (blood) and other tissues (e.g. secondary lymphoid tissues). The above diagram shows the immature Double Negative (CD4-/CD8-) T-cell entering the thymus at the corticomedullary junction to eventually progess in the cortex to become Double Positive (CD4+/CD8+) T-cells that undergo further maturation to eventually enter the medullary portion of the thymus as CD4+/CD8- or CD4-/CD8+ (Single Positive) T-cells.

In summary: The T-cells start as CD4-/CD8-(Double Negative), then become CD4+/CD8+ (Double Positive), and following a MHC induced positive and negative selection process, they eventually become mature CD4+/CD8- or CD4-/CD8+ (Single Positive) T-cells which will enter blood and various tissues. Note that in contrast to the B-cells which start their early maturation in the bone marrow, T-cells start their maturation process in the thymus. Mnemonic is "B" for B-cells and Bone marrow and "T" for T-cells and thymus. Within one T-cell maturation scheme, the T-cell receptor (TCR) gene rearrangement occurs in a predictable ordered fashion with the γ (gamma) and δ (delta) genes rearranging before the α (alpha) and β (beta) genes in the double negative stage of the T-cells. The γ/δ rearrangements that do not give rise to functional γ/δ TCR proteins will then undergo α and β gene rearrangement to ultimately give rise to a functional α/β type TCR protein which comprises the vast majority Tf the TCR proteins.

🔹 T-cell Lymphoblastic Leukemia/Lymphoma

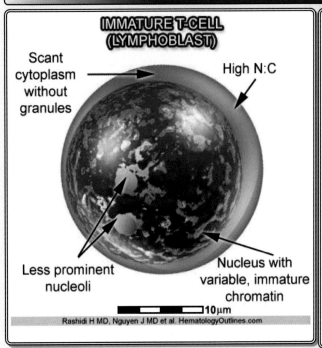

IMMATURE T-CELL (LYMPHOBLAST)

Scant cytoplasm without granules

High N:C

Less prominent nucleoli

Nucleus with variable, immature chromatin

10μm

Rashidi H MD, Nguyen J MD et al. HematologyOutlines.com

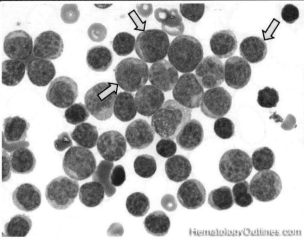

The majority of the cells shown here are immature and consistent with blasts (yellow arrows). Note the scattered smaller mature lymphocytes (minority of cells) in the background.

🔬 Microscopic Features
- 3-4X larger than a mature RBC
- *High nuclear-to-cytoplasmic ratio*
- Round nucleus with immature chromatin (not clumped) and prominent nucleoli
- Cytoplasm is scant, light blue in color and lacks granules

⚠ Frequency in Tissues
- Peripheral Blood: ⊘ None
- Bone Marrow: ⊘ None
- Lymph Node: ⊘ None

↔ May Resemble
- B-lymphoblast {p. 65}
- Myeloblast {p. 21}
- Pronormoblast {p. 9}
- Immature B-cell (hematogone) {p. 62}
- Monoblast {p. 38}
- Prolymphocyte
- Reactive Lymphocyte {p. 137}

Dx Differential Diagnoses
- T-Lymphoblastic leukemia/lymphoma (T-ALL)
- B-Lymphoblastic leukemia/lymphoma (B-ALL)
- Acute myeloid leukemia
- Immature thymic T-cells (e.g. in a thymoma, etc.)

⚙ Classic Immunophenotype
- Cortical:
  - CD4 ➕ and CD8 ➕
  - CD1a ➕, TdT ➕, and CD34 ➕
  - CD2 ➕ / CD5 ➕ / CD7 ➕
  - sCD3 ➕
- Precortical:
  - CD4 ➖, CD8 ➖, and CD19 ➖
  - TdT ➕ / ➖ and CD34 ➕ / ➖
  - CD2 ➕ / ➖ ,CD3 ➕ / ➖, CD5 ➕ / ➖, CD7 ➕ / ➖

Miscellaneous: This neoplasm can arise from the thymus (anterior mediastinum). Remember the mnemonic for anterior mediastinal lesions/masses: 4 Ts (Thymoma, Terrible lymphoma such as T-lymphoblastic lymphoma, Thyroid neoplasms, and Teratoma or other germ cell neoplasms).

Secondary Lymphoid Tissues: Overview Mindmap

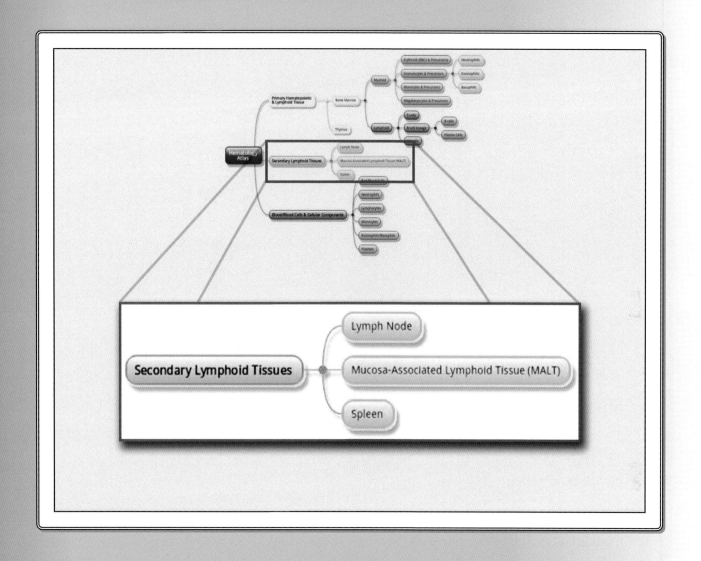

Normal Lymph Node Diagram

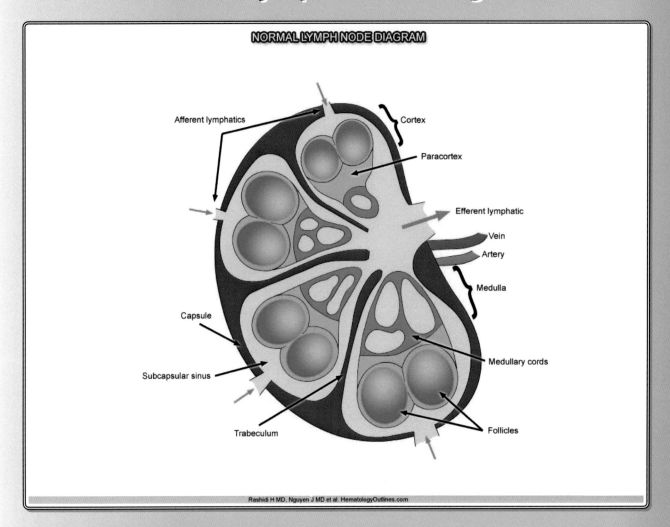

As opposed to the mucosa associated lymphoid tissue, the lymph node is encapsulated. The lymph node can be divided into two main parts, the cortex and the medulla. The follicles (primary and secondary follicles) are predominantly within the cortex. The B-cells are mainly in the follicles while the T-cells are predominantly found in the interfollicular areas.

B-cell Maturation in Lymph Node Diagram

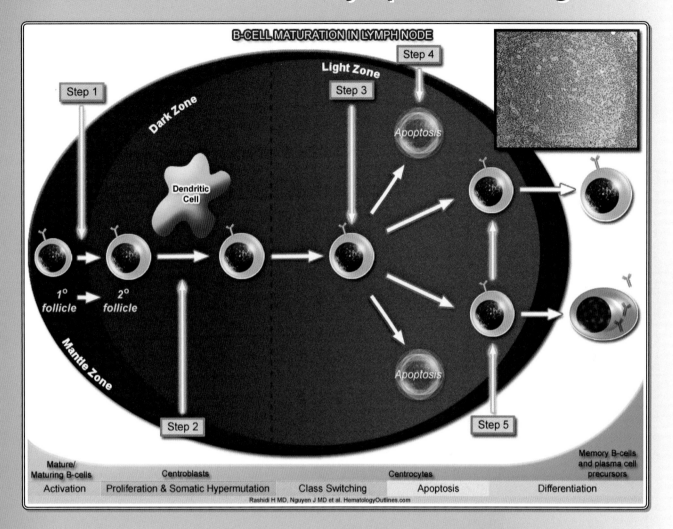

Steps involved in completing B-cell maturation within the germinal center of secondary follicles:

- **Step 1.** Antigen stimulation changes the primary follicle to a secondary follicle with a germinal center.
- **Step 2.** B cells proliferate as centroblasts and somatic hypermutation occurs.
- **Step 3.** Centroblasts give rise to centrocytes and interact with follicular dendritic cells.
- **Step 4.** If a B cell has mutated to have an antibody with more affinity to an antigen, it survives. Otherwise, it undergoes apoptosis.
- **Step 5.** Interaction with helper T cells happens here. Class switching occurs and the B cells become either a plasma cells or memory B cells.

🔥 Normal Lymph Node

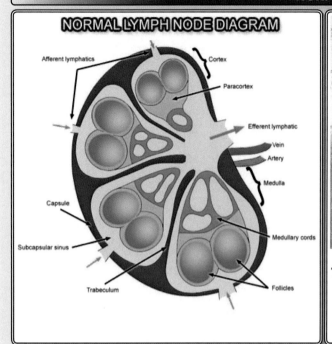

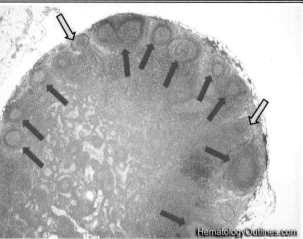

The yellow arrows point to the primary follicles, and the red arrows point to the secondary follicles.

🔬 Microscopic Features
- An encapsulated lymphoid tissue (as opposed to Mucosa Associated Lymphoid Tissue, also known as MALT)
- *Comprised of follicles (primary and secondary) and interfollicular areas*
- B-cells mostly reside in the follicles while T-cells mostly reside in between the follicles (interfollicular areas)
- Most of the follicles are located within the cortex

⚠ Frequency in Tissues
- Peripheral Blood: N/A
- Bone Marrow: N/A
- Lymph Node: N/A

↔ May Resemble
- Non-neoplastic lymphadenitis
- Follicular Lymphoma {p. 79}

ᴰx Differential Diagnoses
- Reactive lymphoid hyperplasia
- Infectious
- Lymphadenitis
- Follicular lymphoma

⚙ Classic Immunophenotype
- "T"-cells = "Tiny" CDs: CD2, CD3, CD4, CD5, CD7, CD8
- "B"-cells = "Bigger" CDs: CD19, CD20, CD22

Miscellaneous: In a normal lymph, the primary follicles (not antigen stimulated and without a germinal center) and secondary follicles (antigen stimulated with a germinal center) are where most B-cell reside. The interfollicular areas (between follicles) are where most T-cells reside.

📓**Note**: In summary, B-cells mostly reside in the follicles while T-cells mostly reside in between the follicles (interfollicular areas).

🔥 GI Tract (Non-Gastric, e.g. Small Bowel): Mucosa Associated Lymphoid Tissue (MALT)

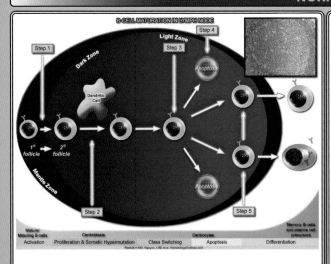

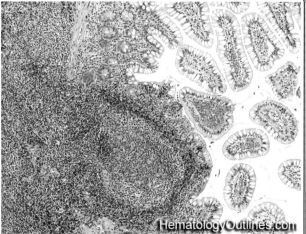

This is a diagram of B-cell maturation seen in germinal centers found within the mucosa associated lymphoid tissue.

The right side shows the intestinal mucosa and the left side shows the mucosa associated lymphoid tissue with a germinal center in the middle.

🔬 Microscopic Features
- *Normal lymphoid tissue that is associated with certain mucosal sites such as the small intestinal Peyer's patches in contrast to normal lymph nodes; these Mucosa Associated Lymphoid Tissue, or MALT, are not encapsulated*
- Similar to lymph nodes, they are comprised of follicles (primary and secondary) and interfollicular areas
- The primary follicles (not antigen stimulated and lacks a germinal center) and secondary follicles (antigen stimulated with a germinal center in the middle) are the B-cell zones. The interfollicular (between follicles) areas are the T-cell zones.

⚠️ Frequency in Tissues
- Peripheral Blood: N/A
- Bone Marrow: N/A
- Lymph Node: N/A

↔️ May Resemble
- Mantle Cell Lymphoma {p. 81}
- MALT Lymphoma {p. 84}
- Normal Spleen {p. 85}
- Normal reactive lymph node

Dx Differential Diagnoses
- Follicular lymphoma
- Mantle cell lymphoma
- Marginal zone lymphoma
- Reactive lymphoid hyperplasia

⚙️ Classic Immunophenotype
- 'T'-cells = 'Tiny' CDs: CD2, CD3, CD4, CD5, CD7, CD8
- 'B'-cells = 'Bigger' CDs: CD19, CD20, CD22

Miscellaneous: Similar to lymph nodes and the spleen, the primary follicles (not antigen stimulated and lacks a germinal center) and secondary follicles (antigen stimulated with a germinal center in the middle) are the B-cell zones and the interfollicular (between follicles) areas are the T-cell zones.

🩸 Small Lymphocytic Lymphoma

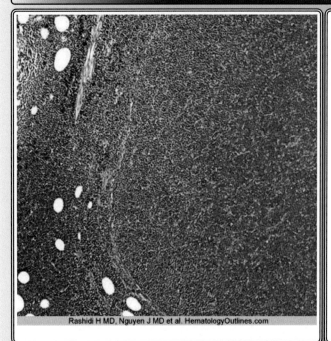

Rashidi H MD, Nguyen J MD et al. HematologyOutlines.com

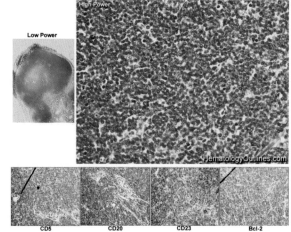

The field of view shows involvement by increased number of small to intermediate-sized lymphocytes that are CD5+, CD23+. CD20+, and Bcl-2+.

🔬 Microscopic Features
- *Increased number of small to intermediate-sized lymphocytes diffusely involving the lymph node*
- Scattered background pseudofollicles are also sometimes noted

⚠ Frequency in Tissues
- Peripheral Blood: N/A
- Bone Marrow: N/A
- Lymph Node: N/A

↔ May Resemble
- Non-neoplastic reactive lymph node
- Mantle Cell Lymphoma {p. 81}
- Follicular Lymphoma {p. 79}

ᴅx Differential Diagnoses
- Non-neoplastic reactive lymph node
- Follicular lymphoma
- Mantle cell lymphoma
- Burkitt Lymphoma
- Diffuse large B-cell lymphoma

⚙ Classic Immunophenotype
- CD19 ➕
- CD20 **dim** ➕
- CD5 ➕
- CD23 ➕
- BCL1 ➖
- Monotypic kappa or lambda **dim** to ➖ surface light chain expression

Miscellaneous: In blood, this disorder is called chronic lymphocytic leukemia (CLL).

📝**Note**: As opposed to CLL which is CD5+/CD23+, mantle cell lymphoma is typically CD5+/CD23-. Also, mantle cell lymphoma is BCL1+ (CyclinD1+) while CLL/SLL is BCL1- (CyclinD1-). Hence, the t(11;14) CyclinD1-IgH translocation is absent in CLL/SLL.

🩸 Follicular Lymphoma

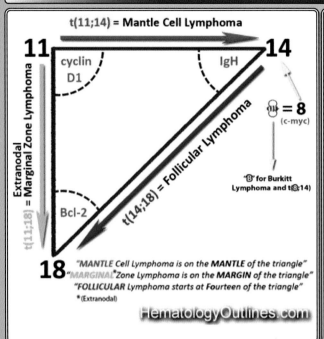

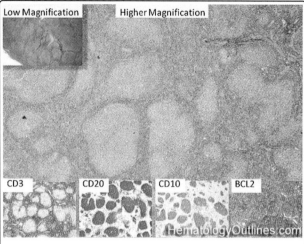

The neoplastic lymphocytes are arranged in a follicular (nodular) pattern and are CD10+, CD20+, and BCL2+. They are negative for CD3.

🔬 Microscopic Features
- The lymph node is usually effaced (closed subcapsular sinus and loss of follicle architecture)
- *The lymphoid tissue is replaced by a back-to-back nodular (follicular) pattern of lymphoid proliferation with a diminished mantle zone*
- The majority of the neoplastic lymphocytes is located in the nodular areas and comprised of small cleaved lymphocytes (centrocytes) with rare scattered larger lymphocytes having multiple peripheralized nucleoli (centroblasts)

⚠️ Frequency in Tissues
- Peripheral Blood: N/A
- Bone Marrow: N/A
- Lymph Node: N/A

↔️ May Resemble
- Non-neoplastic reactive lymph node
- Small Lymphocytic Lymphoma {p. 78}
- Mantle Cell Lymphoma {p. 81}
- Burkitt Lymphoma {p. 82}

Dx Differential Diagnoses
- Non-neoplastic reactive lymph node
- Small lymphocytic lymphoma
- Mantle cell lymphoma
- Burkitt lymphoma
- Diffuse large B-cell lymphoma

⚙️ Classic Immunophenotype
- CD19 ➕ and CD20 ➕
- CD10 ➕
- BCL6 ➕
- BCL2 ➕
- CD5 ➖

Miscellaneous: Mantle cell lymphoma is associated with t(14;18) IgH:BCL2 genes, as opposed to Burkitt lymphoma which is also CD10+ but with a Ki67 of ~100%. The Ki67 (proliferative index) in most follicular lymphomas is much lower. Additionally, similar to other low grade lymphomas, the BCL2 protein (anti-apoptotic protein and not the gene) is typically overexpressed in most follicular lymphomas. In contrast, high grade lymphomas with increased apoptotic cells, such as Burkitt lymphoma, usually lack expression of the BCL2 protein.

⬥ Diffuse Large B-cell Lymphoma

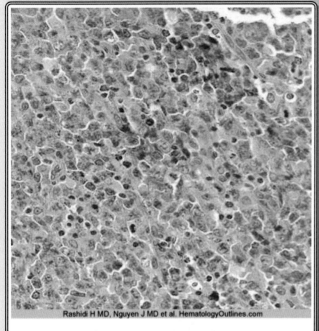

Rashidi H MD, Nguyen J MD et al. HematologyOutlines.com

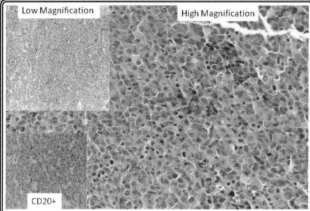

Low Magnification

High Magnification

CD20+

HematologyOutlines.com

Sheets of large abnormal lymphocytes that are CD20+ are seen in this image and the one to the left.

⚗ Microscopic Features
- *Sheets or clusters of large (>2.5X the size of a mature lymphocyte or equal or greater than the size of a histiocyte) abnormal lymphocytes involving lymph node or other tissue*
- As the name suggests, the abnormal lymphocytes diffusely infiltrate the involved tissue (typically lacks a nodular/follicular pattern of growth)

⚠ Frequency in Tissues
- Peripheral Blood: N/A
- Bone Marrow: N/A
- Lymph Node: N/A

↔ May Resemble
- Burkitt Lymphoma {p. 82}
- Small Lymphocytic Lymphoma {p. 78}
- Mantle Cell Lymphoma {p. 81}
- Follicular Lymphoma {p. 79}
- Non-neoplastic reactive lymph node
- Carcinoma
- Melanoma

ᴰx Differential Diagnoses
- Mantle cell lymphoma (blastoid variant)
- Follicular lymphoma (high grade, e.g. 3B)
- Burkitt lymphoma
- Small lymphocytic lymphoma
- Mantle cell lymphoma
- Non-neoplastic reactive lymph node
- Hodgkin lymphoma

✿ Classic Immunophenotype
- CD19 ➕
- CD20 ➕
- CD10 ➕ (germinal center phenotype)
- CD10 ➖ /BCL6 ➖ /MUM1 ➕ (non-germinal center phenotype)

Miscellaneous: Germinal center phenotype (CD10+) has better prognosis (usually responds better to R-CHOP chemotherapy treatment). Diffuse large B-cell lymphoma is diverse in that many have variable morphology (some with prominent nucleoli, some with high mitotic rate, etc.) and many present as mass lesions.

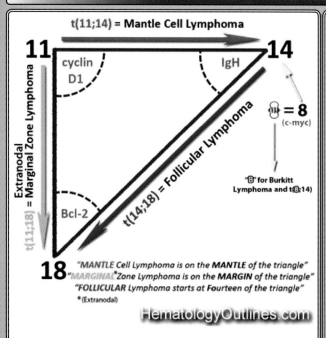

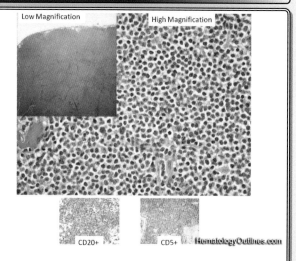

The lymph node above is effaced and replaced by a diffuse lymphoid proliferation of small to intermediate-sized notched lymphocytes that are CD5+ and CD20+.

🔬 Microscopic Features
- The lymph node is usually effaced (closed subcapsular sinus and loss of follicle architecture)
- *The lymphoid tissue is replaced by usually a diffuse lymphoid proliferation of small to intermediate-sized notched lymphocytes (the abnormal lymphocytes have irregular nuclear membranes)*

⚠ Frequency in Tissues
- Peripheral Blood: N/A
- Bone Marrow: N/A
- Lymph Node: N/A

↔ May Resemble
- Non-neoplastic reactive lymph node
- Small Lymphocytic Lymphoma {p. 78}
- Follicular Lymphoma {p. 79} (especially the nodular variant of mantle cell lymphoma)

Dx Differential Diagnoses
- Non-neoplastic reactive lymph node
- Small lymphocytic lymphoma
- Follicular lymphoma (especially the nodular variant of Mantle cell lymphoma)
- Burkitt lymphoma
- Diffuse large B-cell lymphoma

⚙ Classic Immunophenotype
- CD19 ➕
- CD20 ➕
- CD5 ➕
- CD23 ➖
- BCL1 ➕ (CyclinD1 ➕)

Miscellaneous: BCL1+ (Cyclin D1+) is associated with t(11;14) CyclinD1:IgH genes.

Note: Lymphomatoid polyposis is "mantle cell lymphoma" involving the colon and may resemble a polyp.

Note: As opposed to CLL which is CD5+/CD23+, mantle cell lymphoma is typically CD5+/CD23-.

⬥ Burkitt Lymphoma

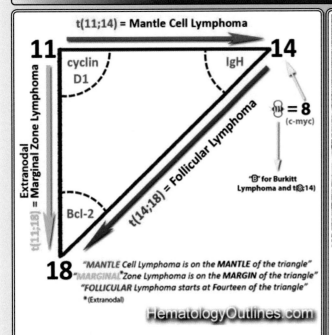

t(11;14) = Mantle Cell Lymphoma

11 cyclin D1 **14** IgH

Extranodal = Marginal Zone Lymphoma

t(11;18)

Bcl-2

t(14;18) = Follicular Lymphoma

🔬 = **8** (c-myc)

"Ⓑ" for Burkitt Lymphoma and t(8;14)

18

"*MANTLE* Cell Lymphoma is on the **MANTLE** of the triangle"
"*MARGINAL* Zone Lymphoma is on the **MARGIN** of the triangle"
"*FOLLICULAR* Lymphoma starts at Fourteen of the triangle"
* (Extranodal)

HematologyOutlines.com

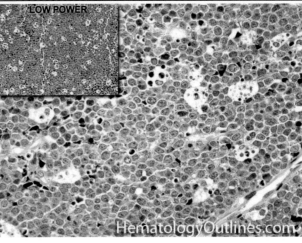

LOW POWER

HematologyOutlines.com

The above depicts a "starry-sky" pattern with a diffuse lymphoid proliferation of intermediate sized lymphocytes, apoptotic cells, and a very high mitotic rate.

🔬 Microscopic Features
- *"Starry Sky" pattern due to many background apoptotic cells*
- The lymph node is usually effaced (closed subcapsular sinus and loss of follicle architecture)
- The normal lymphoid tissue is replaced by a diffuse lymphoid proliferation of intermediate sized lymphocytes with a very high mitotic rate

⚠ Frequency in Tissues
- Peripheral Blood: N/A
- Bone Marrow: N/A
- Lymph Node: N/A

↔ May Resemble
- Diffuse Large B-cell Lymphoma {p. 80}
- Small Lymphocytic Lymphoma {p. 78}
- Mantle Cell Lymphoma {p. 81}
- Non-neoplastic reactive lymph node

ᴅx Differential Diagnoses
- Non-neoplastic reactive lymph node
- Small lymphocytic lymphoma
- Mantle cell lymphoma
- Diffuse large B-cell lymphoma
- Follicular lymphoma

⚙ Classic Immunophenotype
- CD19 ⊞
- CD20 ⊞
- CD10 ⊞
- BCL2 ⊟
- CD5 ⊟
- Ki67 proliferation index is nearly 100%

Miscellaneous: Burkitt lymphoma is associated with t(8;14) c-MYC;IgH genes. It is less commonly associated with other translocations including the light chains (kappa or lambda): t(2;8) or t(8;22).

💧 ALK+ Anaplastic Large Cell Lymphoma

ABNORMAL

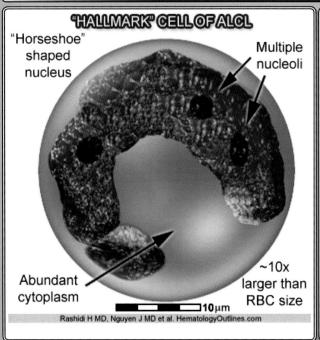

"HALLMARK" CELL OF ALCL

"Horseshoe" shaped nucleus

Multiple nucleoli

Abundant cytoplasm

~10x larger than RBC size

10μm

Rashidi H MD, Nguyen J MD et al. HematologyOutlines.com

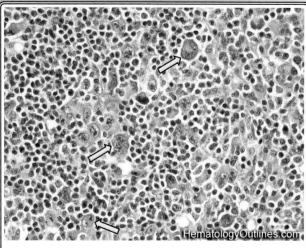

The arrows highlight the "hallmark" cells.

HematologyOutlines.com

🔬 Microscopic Features
- Sheets or clusters of large (>2.5X the size of a mature lymphocyte or equal or greater than the size of a histiocyte) abnormal lymphocytes usually involving lymph node but may involve other tissue
- *Anaplastic Large Cell Lymphoma (ALCL) usually has horseshoe-shaped large abnormal cells known as "hallmark cells"*
- ALCL typically involves the lymph node sinuses but it may have a diffuse pattern of growth as well

⚠️ Frequency in Tissues
- Peripheral Blood: N/A
- Bone Marrow: N/A
- Lymph Node: N/A

↔️ May Resemble
- RS cells (Hodgkin lymphoma, see in Glossary)
- Non-neoplastic reactive lymph node
- Diffuse Large B-cell Lymphoma {p. 80}
- Burkitt Lymphoma {p. 82}
- Small Lymphocytic Lymphoma {p. 78}
- Mantle Cell Lymphoma {p. 81}
- Follicular Lymphoma {p. 79}
- Carcinoma
- Melanoma

Dx Differential Diagnoses
- Hodgkin lymphoma
- Diffuse large B-cell lymphoma
- Mantle cell lymphoma (blastoid variant)
- Follicular lymphoma (high grade, e.g. 3B)
- Burkitt lymphoma
- Small lymphocytic lymphoma
- Non-neoplastic reactive lymph node

⚙️ Classic Immunophenotype
- CD3 ➕ / ➖
- CD2 ➕ / ➖, CD5 ➕ / ➖, CD7 ➕ / ➖
- CD30 ➕
- ALK ➕
- PAX5 ➖ and CD20 ➖

Miscellaneous: Most are associated with the t(2;5) ALK1-NPM translocation, especially if the ALK IHC staining pattern shows a nuclear and cytoplasmic staining pattern.

💧 MALT Lymphoma (e.g. Gastric)

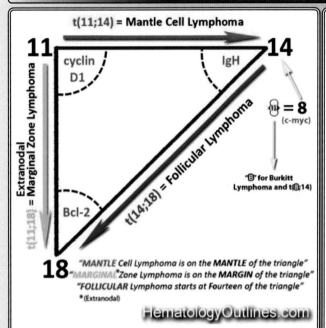

Note: If t(11;18) is present then the genes are NOT cyclin D1 and Bcl-2, but instead involve the AP12 and MLT1 genes.

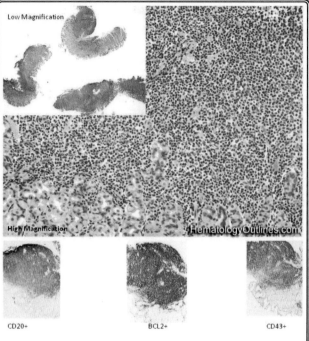

CD20+   BCL2+   CD43+

These lymphoma cells are small in size and typically low-grade (low Ki-67 and Bcl-2+).

🔬 Microscopic Features
- *Small- to intermediate-sized lymphocytes (many with monocytoid features which show increased amount of cytoplasm)*
- Lymphoepithelial lesions (neoplastic lymphocytes infiltrating and destroying the epithelial glandular tissue)

⚠️ Frequency in Tissues
- Peripheral Blood: ⊘ None
- Bone Marrow: ⊘ None
- Lymph Node: ⊘ None

↔ May Resemble
- H. pylori gastritis
- Follicular Lymphoma {p. 79}
- Diffuse Large B-cell Lymphoma {p. 80}
- Lymphoplasmacytic lymphoma
- Small Lymphocytic Lymphoma {p. 78}
- Mantle Cell Lymphoma {p. 81}

Dx Differential Diagnoses
- Infection (specifically H. Pylori in stomach)
- Mantle cell lymphoma
- Follicular lymphoma
- Lymphoplasmacytic lymphoma
- Diffuse large B-cell lymphoma

⚙ Classic Immunophenotype
- CD19 ➕ and CD20 ➕
- Bcl-2 ➕
- CD5 ➖, CD10 ➖, CD23 ➖
- CD43 ➕/➖
- BCL1 ➖
- Low Ki-67

Miscellaneous: Gastric MALT lymphoma is usually associated with H. pylori.

Note: Extranodal MALT lymphomas are more common in locations that usually lack normal MALT lymphoid tissue (e.g. gastric).

NORMAL

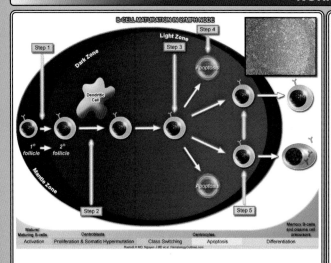

This is a diagram of B-cell maturation seen in germinal centers found within the splenic white pulp.

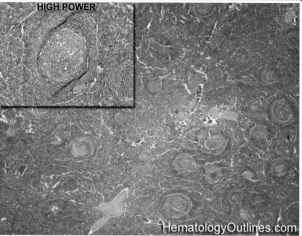

The nodular lymphoid areas represent the white pulp while the intervening areas are the red pulp. The high power inset shows a reactive follicle comprising of the central germinal center surrounded by the mantle zone and the outermost marginal zone areas.

🔬 Microscopic Features
- ***Spleen is divided into 2 main zones: red pulp and white pulp***
- The white pulp contains the lymphoid cells and appears as small blue/purple aggregates of lymphoid tissue
- The red pulp contains the sinusoids along with scattered hematopoietic cells and appears red

⚠ Frequency in Tissues
- Peripheral Blood: N/A
- Bone Marrow: N/A
- Lymph Node: N/A

↔ May Resemble
- Normal Lymph Node {p. 76}
- Normal Mucosa Associated Lymphoid Tissue (MALT) {p. 77}

ᴰx Differential Diagnoses
- Reactive lymphoid hyperplasia
- Infection
- Splenic marginal zone lymphoma
- Hairy cell leukemia
- Follicular lymphoma

⚙ Classic Immunophenotype
- "T"-cells = "Tiny" CDs: CD2, CD3, CD4 ➕ / ➖, CD5, CD7, CD8 ➕ / ➖
- "B"-cells = "Bigger" CDs: CD19, CD20, CD22

Miscellaneous: In splenic marginal zone lymphoma, the neoplastic cells involve the white pulp areas of the spleen (in contrast to hairy cell leukemia which involves the red pulp areas).

B-cell Maturation in Spleen Diagram

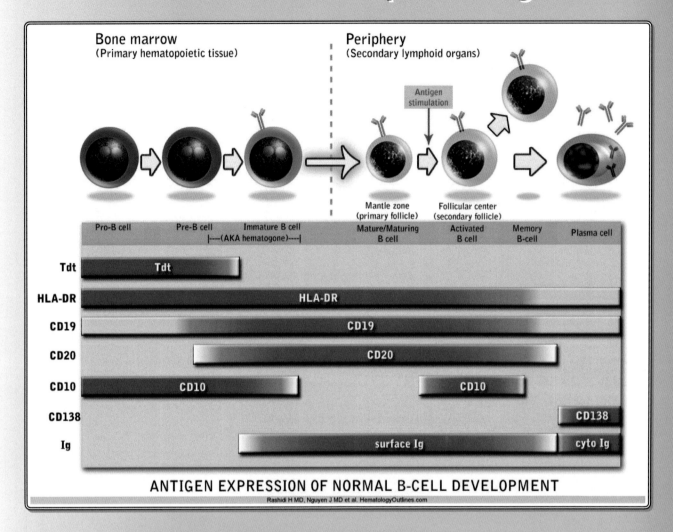

Bone marrow (Primary hematopoietic tissue)

Periphery (Secondary lymphoid organs)

Antigen stimulation

Mantle zone (primary follicle)

Follicular center (secondary follicle)

	Pro-B cell	Pre-B cell	Immature B cell |----(AKA hematogone)----|	Mature/Maturing B cell	Activated B cell	Memory B-cell	Plasma cell
Tdt	Tdt					
HLA-DR	HLA-DR					
CD19	CD19					
CD20		CD20				
CD10	CD10			CD10		
CD138						CD138
Ig			surface Ig			cyto Ig

ANTIGEN EXPRESSION OF NORMAL B-CELL DEVELOPMENT

Rashidi H MD, Nguyen J MD et al. HematologyOutlines.com

B-cell maturation starts with B-cell precursors in the bone marrow. These precursors progress to becoming hematogones (various stages of immature B-cells in the bone marrow) and then become early maturing B-cells in the bone marrow. These early maturing B-cells then leave the bone marrow and end up in secondary lymphoid tissues (e.g. Lymph nodes, Mucosa Associated Lymphoid Tissue or Spleen) where they finish their maturation process upon antigen stimulation (During pre-antigen stimulation, these B-cells are predominantly in primary follicles and upon antigen stimulation they enter the germinal center of secondary follicles where somatic hypermutation and class switching occurs that eventually give rise to memory B-cells and plasma cells).

As opposed to B-cells that have surface bound immunoglobulins (Ig), the Ig of plasma cells are cytoplasmic because they are made to be secreted. Additionally, as opposed to both B-cells and T-cells which circulate in the peripheral blood, plasma cells are usually absent in blood.

Note: All B-cells express some level of CD19 and as antigen presenting cells they would be expected to also express MHC class II molecules which explains the expression of HLA-DR (a MHC class II) on all B-cells (from early B-cells to plasma cells).

⬥ Hairy Cell Leukemia

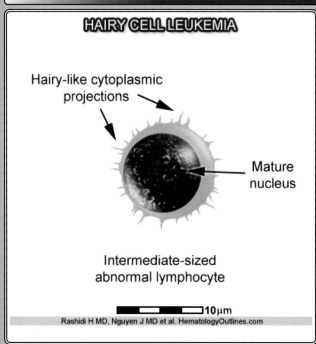

HAIRY CELL LEUKEMIA

Hairy-like cytoplasmic projections

Mature nucleus

Intermediate-sized abnormal lymphocyte

▮▮▮▮▮▮▮10µm

Rashidi H MD, Nguyen J MD et al. HematologyOutlines.com

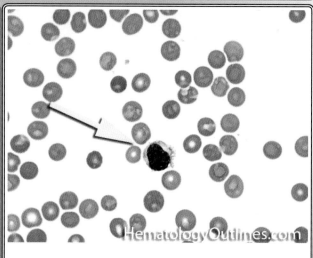

The arrow points to the hairy cell. It has a nucleus which is slightly larger than the RBCs with a fair amount of cytoplasm with hair-like projections.

🔬 Microscopic Features
- ***Peripheral blood smear shows lymphocytes with hair-like cytoplasmic projections***
- Abnormal lymphocytes with hair-like projections are intermediate in size
- Lacks a nucleolus but some may have a small nucleolus
- The neoplastic cells typically involve the red pulp areas of the spleen (as opposed to splenic marginal zone lymphoma which involves the white pulp)

⚠ Frequency in Tissues
- Peripheral Blood: ⊘ None
- Bone Marrow: ⊘ None
- Lymph Node: ⊘ None

↔ May Resemble
- Splenic Marginal Zone Lymphoma {p. 88}
- Reactive Lymphocyte {p. 137}
- Chronic Lymphocytic Leukemia (CLL) {p. 139}

Dx Differential Diagnoses
- Splenic marginal zone lymphoma
- Reactive lymphocytosis
- Chronic lymphocytic leukemia
- Lymphoplasmacytic lymphoma

⚙ Classic Immunophenotype
- CD19 ⊞ and CD20 ⊞
- CD23 ⊖
- CD5 ⊖
- CD10 ⊖
- CD103 ⊞
- CD11c ⊞
- CD25 ⊞
- Annexin A1 ⊞

Miscellaneous: Many cases present with splenomegaly, cytopenia or pancytopenia (many with monocytopenia), and a dry bone marrow aspirate (dry tap). Most cases also carry the BRAF V600E mutation.

⬤ Splenic Marginal Zone Lymphoma

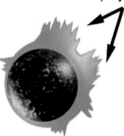

SPLENIC MARGINAL ZONE LYMPHOMA

Villous cytoplasmic projections

Abnormal lymphocytes are intermediate in size

10μm

Rashidi H MD, Nguyen J MD et al. HematologyOutlines.com

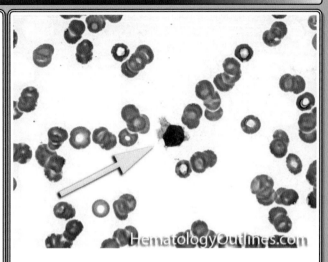

HematologyOutlines.com

The abnormal cells may show villous cytoplasmic projections as indicated by the yellow arrow.

🔬 Microscopic Features
- *Peripheral blood smear shows lymphocytes with villous cytoplasmic projections (may resemble hair-like projections as seen in hairy cell leukemia)*
- Lymphocytes with villous-like projections are intermediate in size
- Lacks a prominent nucleolus

⚠ Frequency in Tissues
- Peripheral Blood: ⊘ None
- Bone Marrow: ⊘ None
- Lymph Node: ⊘ None

↔ May Resemble
- Hairy Cell Leukemia {p. 141}
- Reactive Lymphocyte {p. 137}
- Chronic Lymphocytic Leukemia (CLL) {p. 139}

Dx Differential Diagnoses
- Hairy cell leukemia
- Reactive lymphocytosis
- Chronic lymphocytic leukemia (CLL)

⚙ Classic Immunophenotype
- CD19 ➕ and CD20 ➕
- CD23 ➖
- CD5 ➖
- CD10 ➖
- CD11c ➖
- CD43 ➕/➖
- CD103 ➖
- CD25 ➖
- Annexin A1 ➖

Miscellaneous: The neoplastic cells typically involve the white pulp areas of the spleen (in contrast to hairy cell leukemia which involves the red pulp).

Peripheral Blood: Overview Mindmap

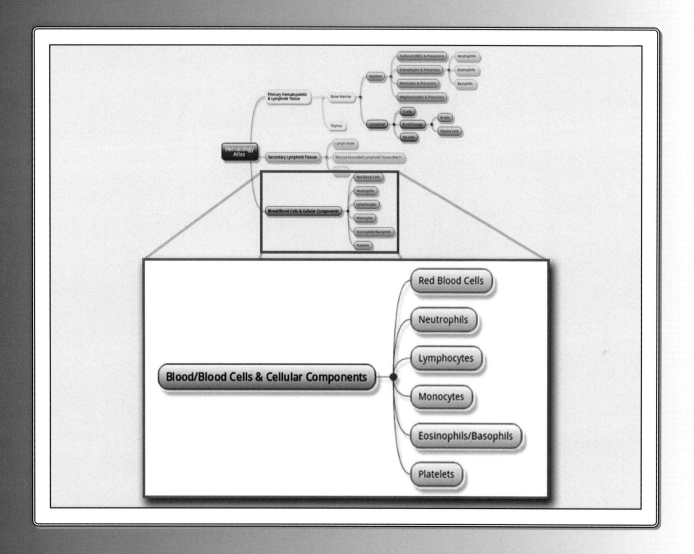

Erythrocyte (RBC) Maturation Diagram

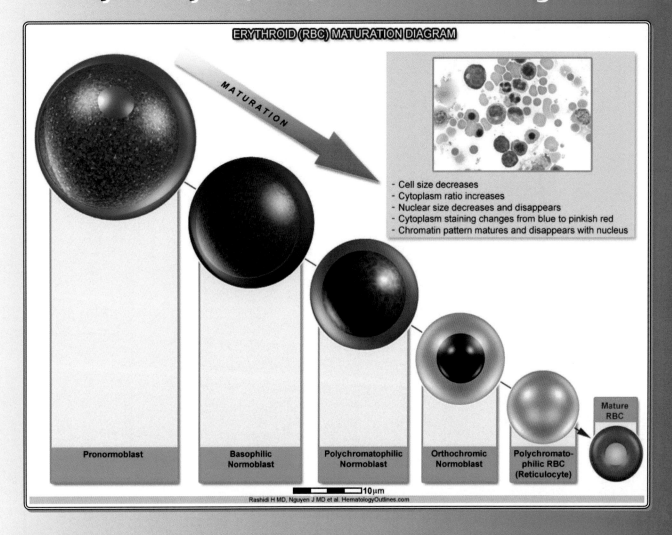

ERYTHROID (RBC) MATURATION DIAGRAM

MATURATION

- Cell size decreases
- Cytoplasm ratio increases
- Nuclear size decreases and disappears
- Cytoplasm staining changes from blue to pinkish red
- Chromatin pattern matures and disappears with nucleus

| Pronormoblast | Basophilic Normoblast | Polychromatophilic Normoblast | Orthochromic Normoblast | Polychromato-philic RBC (Reticulocyte) | Mature RBC |

10 µm

Rashidi H MD, Nguyen J MD et al. HematologyOutlines.com

The goal of the erythroid maturation process is to give rise to the mature red blood cell (RBC). Ultimately this is accomplished by losing its nucleus and increasing its hemoglobin content to maximize the RBC's oxygen carrying capacity. Understanding this normal maturation process is essential in understanding RBC disorders.

NORMAL

NORMAL MATURE RED BLOOD CELL

Central pallor is
1/3 diameter

⟷

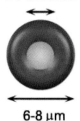

6-8 μm

⟷

━━━━━━━━10μm

Rashidi, MD & Nguyen, MD et al. HematologyOutlines.com

central pallor is
~1/3 diameter

HematologyOutlines.com

Peripheral smear
Laying flat, the red blood cell can be equally divided
into thirds by the size of the central pallor.

🔬 Microscopic Features
- Size 6-8 μm, slightly smaller than a mature lymphocyte
- *Lacks a nucleus*
- Cytoplasm is pink-orange in color with a central pallor
- Central pallor is 1/3 the diameter

⚠ Frequency in Tissues
- Peripheral blood: ● Many
- Bone marrow: ● Many
- Lymphoid tissue: ◉ Some

↔ May Resemble
- Polychromatophilic RBC {p. 92}
- Macrocytic RBC {p. 95}
- Microcytic RBC {p. 94}
- Giant Platelet {p. 155}

Dx Differential Diagnoses
- ↑ Increased in:
  - Reactive erythroid hyperplasia
  - Post-erythropoietin therapy
  - Polycythemia vera

⚙ Classic Immunophenotype
- CD45 ⊖
- CD117 ⊖
- CD235a (Glycophorin A) ⊞
- Hemoglobin ⊞
- CD71 ⊖

Miscellaneous: Normal mature RBCs are normocytic (MCV 80-100μm) and normochromic (1/3 central pallor). Its main function is to carry oxygen via its hemoglobin molecules.

Note: As erythroid precursors mature, the color of their cytoplasm changes from blue to gray to red-orange (this is due to the increase in the number of hemoglobin molecules within the red blood cells as they mature). Additionally, the nucleus of the red blood cell will become more dense as it matures, eventually excreting from the cell forming the mature red blood cell.

🩸 Polychromatophilic RBC

POLYCHROMATOPHILIC RED BLOOD CELL (RETICULOCYTE WITH SPECIAL STAIN)

Called a reticulocyte when precipitated RNA can be highlighted with supravital stain

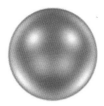

Lacks a nucleus

10μm

Rashidi H MD, Nguyen J MD et al. HematologyOutlines.com

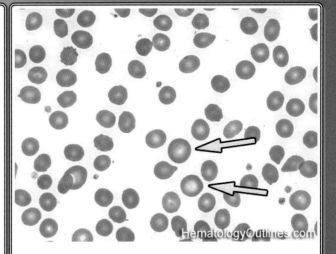

HematologyOutlines.com

Note the slightly larger RBCs by the yellow arrows. These polychromatophilic RBCs are slightly less mature and have a greyish color (due to RNA).

🔬 Microscopic Features
- **Slightly larger than normal mature RBCs**
- Lacks a nucleus
- Cytoplasm is greyish-orange in color (since it is less mature than a normal mature RBC)

⚠ Frequency in Tissues
- Peripheral Blood: 1-2%
- Bone Marrow: 🔆 Scattered
- Lymph Node: ○ Rare to ⊘ None

↔ May Resemble
- With normal stain (not supravital) may resemble:
  ○ Mature RBC {p. 91}
  ○ Macrocytic RBC {p. 95}
  ○ Giant Platelet {p. 155} (especially if hypogranular)
- Reticulocyte (with supravital stain) may resemble:
  ○ Heinz Bodies {p. 110}
  ○ RBC with stain artifact

ᴰˣ Differential Diagnoses
- ↑ Increased in:
  ○ In response to some anemias (e.g. hemolytic anemia or blood loss)
  ○ Reactive erythroid hyperplasia
  ○ Post erythropoeitin therapy
  ○ Polycythemia vera
  ○ May be increased in newborns

⚙ Classic Immunophenotype
- Hemoglobin ➕
- CD45 ➖
- CD117 ➖
- CD235a (Glycophorin A) ➕
- CD71 ➖

Miscellaneous: A polychromatophilic red blood cell is called a reticulocyte when supravital stain highlights the precipitated RNA.

Abnormal Red blood Cell Morphologies

Abnormal RBC Morphology	Cartoon Image	May be associated with
Microcytic RBC		Pyridoxine deficiency Thalassemia Iron deficiency anemia Chronic disease anemia (sometimes) Sideroblastic anemia (sometimes)
Macrocytic RBC		Vitamin B12 or Folate deficiency Liver Disease MDS Chemotherapy (e.g. methotrexate)
Spurr Cell RBC (Acanthocyte)		Abetalipoproteinemia Liver disease McLeod blood group phenotype Post-splenectomy Etc.
Burr Cell RBC (Echinocyte)		Artifact Uremia Liver disease Etc.
Schistocyte		Microangiopathic Hemolytic Anemia Mechanical valve induced Etc.
Bite Cell RBC		G6PD deficiency Unstable hemoglobin disorders Oxidative drugs
Elliptocyte		Hereditary elliptocytosis Severe iron deficiency anemia
Spherocyte		Hereditary spherocytosis Autoimmune hemolytic anemia
Stomatocyte		Hereditary stomatocytosis Liver disease
Target Cell RBC		Thalassemia Hemoglobinopathies Post-splenectomy Liver disease Artifact
Sickle Cell RBC		Hemoglobin SS disease Hemoglobin SC disease Hemoglobin SD disease S-beta thalassemia
Teardrop		Myelofibrosis Underlying marrow process/infiltrate Etc.
Hemoglobin C Crystals		Hemoglobin C disease Hemoglobin SC disease
Red Cell Agglutinate		Cold autoimmune hemolytic anemia Paroxysmal cold hemoglobinuria IgM associated lymphoma Multiple myeloma
Rouleaux		Chronic liver disease Malignant lymphoma Multiple myeloma Chronic inflammatory diseases

🔵 Microcytic RBC: MCV <80

MICROCYTIC RBC : MCV <80

Normal

10μm

Rashidi H MD, Nguyen J MD et al. HematologyOutlines.com

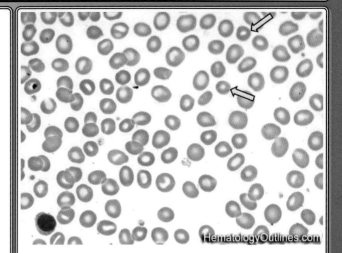

Note the smaller RBCs (microcytic) by the arrows.

🔬 Microscopic Features
- *Slightly smaller than a normal mature RBC which correlates to the MCV of <80 fL*
- Pallor is usually present (as opposed to a microspherocyte)
- Can be hypochromic (central pallor greater than 1/3 of cell diameter), especially in iron deficiency anemia

⚠️ Frequency in Tissues
- Peripheral Blood: ○ Rare to ⊘ None
- Bone Marrow: ○ Rare to ⊘ None
- Lymph Node: ○ Rare to ⊘ None

↔️ May Resemble
- Normal Mature RBC {p. 91}
- Spherocyte {p. 99}

Dx Differential Diagnoses
- Remember the mnemonic "Puny TICS":
  - "Puny" for Pyridoxine (vitamin B6) deficiency
  - "T" for Thalassemia
  - "I" for Iron deficiency anemia
  - "C" for Chronic disease anemia (sometimes): AKA anemia of chronic inflammation/disease
  - "S" for some Sideroblastic anemias (e.g. Lead poisoning)

⚙️ Classic Immunophenotype
- CD45 ⊖
- CD117 ⊖
- CD235a (Glycophorin A) ⊞
- CD71 ⊖

Miscellaneous: Remember the "Puny TICS" mnemonic for microcytic anemias. "Puny" and "TICS" (ticks) are both small, similar to "microcytic" RBCs.

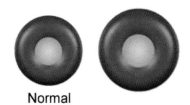

Normal

10µm

Rashidi H MD, Nguyen J MD et al. HematologyOutlines.com

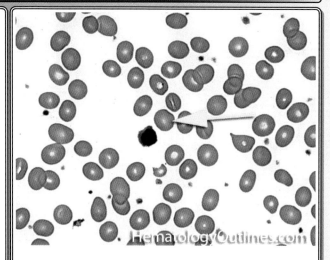

Note the macrocytic RBC by the arrow is larger than the mature lymphocyte nearby.

🔬 Microscopic Features
- ***Slightly larger than a normal mature RBC which correlates to the MCV of >100 fL***
- Round to oval in shape (lacks a nucleus similar to the normal RBC)
- Cytoplasm is pink-orange in color wth a central pallor (similar to a normal RBC)

⚠️ Frequency in Tissues
- Peripheral Blood: ○ Rare to ⊘ None
- Bone Marrow: ○ Rare to ⊘ None
- Lymph Node: ○ Rare to ⊘ None

↔ May Resemble
- Normal Mature RBC {p. 91}
- Polychromatophilic RBC {p. 92}
- Giant Platelet {p. 155} (especially if hypogranular)
- Elliptocyte (ovalocyte) {p. 98}

ᴅx Differential Diagnoses
- Vitamin B12 or folate deficiency
- Chemotherapy (e.g. methotrexate)
- Liver disease
- Thyroid disease
- MDS
- Marked reticulocytosis
- Alcohol
- Certain drugs or infections (e.g. HIV drugs/infection)

⚙️ Classic Immunophenotype
- CD45 ⊖
- CD117 ⊖
- CD235a (Glycophorin A) ⊞
- CD71 ⊖

Miscellaneous: Macrocytic anemia can be divided into megaloblastic (e.g. B12 or folate deficiency) and non-megaloblastic processes. Megaloblastic processes are usually due to defective DNA synthesis while non-megaloblastic ones (e.g. liver disease) cause macrocytic changes through other paths (e.g. lipid deposition in liver disease). Remember, one must rule out vitamin B12 or folate deficiency first.

⬥ Burr cell RBC (Echinocyte)

BURR CELL RBC (ECHINOCYTE)

Evenly distributed,
uniformly sized spicules

|———— 10μm

Rashidi H MD, Nguyen J MD et al. HematologyOutlines.com

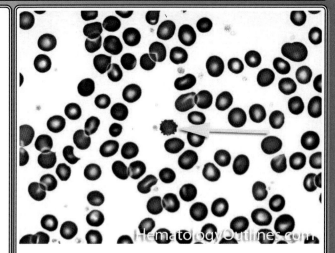

The arrow points at the Burr cell.

🔬 Microscopic Features
- May be smaller or the size as a normal RBC
- *Regular broader-base short blunt projections of the red blood cell membrane*

⚠ Frequency in Tissues
- Peripheral Blood: ○ Rare to ⊘ None
- Bone Marrow: ○ Rare to ⊘ None
- Lymph Node: ○ Rare to ⊘ None

↔ May Resemble
- Spur cell (see in Glossary)
- Schistocyte {p. 100}
- Spherocyte {p. 99}
- Normal Mature RBC {p. 91}

Dx Differential Diagnoses
- Artifact (e.g. older blood specimen)
- Uremia (e.g. chronic renal disease)
- Liver disease
- Hyperlipidemia

⚙ Classic Immunophenotype
- N/A

Miscellaneous: Most often they are due to an artifact of smear preparation. Also one must inquire about the age of the blood sample.

🔵 Bite Cell RBC

BITE CELL RBC

Usually smaller than normal RBC

"Bitten" appearance

━━━━━━━10μm

Rashidi H MD, Nguyen J MD et al. HematologyOutlines.com

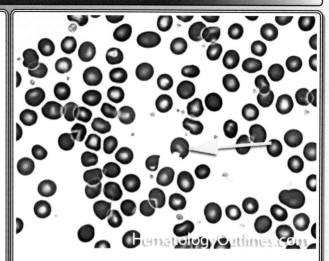

The arrow points at the bite cell.

🔬 Microscopic Features
- Usually slightly smaller than a normal RBC
- *The RBC has a "bitten" appearance (like a bitten apple)*

⚠ Frequency in Tissues
- Peripheral Blood: ○ Rare to ⊘ None
- Bone Marrow: ○ Rare to ⊘ None
- Lymph Node: ○ Rare to ⊘ None

↔ May Resemble
- Schistocyte (Helmet Cell Type) {p. 100}
- Normal Mature RBC {p. 91}

ᴅx Differential Diagnoses
- G6PD deficiency
- Unstable hemoglobin disorders
- Oxidative drug-effect

⚙ Classic Immunophenotype
- N/A

Miscellaneous: Commonly associated with disorders in which precipitated oxidized hemoglobin on the RBC membrane (e.g. Heinz bodies in RBCs of G6PD patients) is removed as they pass through the spleen, ultimately forming a bite-shaped RBC appearance.

🩸 Elliptocyte (Ovalocyte)

ELLIPTOCYTE RBC (OVALOCYTE)

Variable size, but
longer and narrower than normal RBC

Uniform, symmetrical
rod-shapes with rounded ends

10µm

Rashidi H MD, Nguyen J MD et al. HematologyOutlines.com

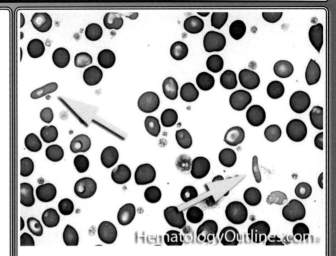

The arrows point at the pencil-shaped elliptocytes.

🔬 Microscopic Features

- Same size or slightly larger than a normal RBC
- *Usually longer and narrower than normal RBC*
- Usually has a central pallor
- Some may be egg-shaped and some may be rod-like (sometimes referred to as pencil cells)

⚠ Frequency in Tissues

- Peripheral Blood: ○ Rare to ⊘ None
- Bone Marrow: ○ Rare to ⊘ None
- Lymph Node: ○ Rare to ⊘ None

↔ May Resemble

- Teardrop Cell {p. 104}
- Macrocytic RBC {p. 95}
- Normal Mature RBC {p. 91}

Dx Differential Diagnoses

- Severe iron deficiency anemia
- Hereditary elliptocytosis
- Thalassemia (sometimes)

⚙ Classic Immunophenotype

- N/A

Miscellaneous: Similar to what is noted in hereditary stomatocytosis and hereditary spherocytosis (HS), hereditary elliptocytosis is also due to an underlying RBC membrane defect. The membrane defect in hereditary elliptocytosis is in many instances due to spectrin, ankyrin, protein 4.1, and glycophorin C.

🌢 Spherocyte

SPHEROCYTE

No central pallor

██████████████10µm

Rashidi H MD, Nguyen J MD et al. HematologyOutlines.com

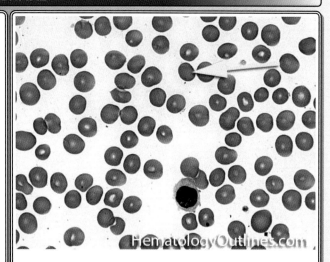

The arrow points to the spherocyte. Notice the lack of a central pallor.

🔬 Microscopic Features
- Usually smaller than a normal RBC
- *MCV may be normal or slightly decreased*
- Very round
- No central pallor

⚠ Frequency in Tissues
- Peripheral Blood: ○ Rare to ⊘ None
- Bone Marrow: ○ Rare to ⊘ None
- Lymph Node: ○ Rare to ⊘ None

↔ May Resemble
- Microcytic RBC {p. 94}
- Polychromatophilic RBC {p. 92}
- Macrocytic RBC {p. 95}
- Normal Mature RBC {p. 91}

Dx Differential Diagnoses
- Hereditary spherocytosis
- Autoimmune hemolytic anemia
- Burn patients
- Artifact

⚙ Classic Immunophenotype
- N/A

Miscellaneous: Similar to hereditary stomatocytosis and hereditary elliptocytosis, hereditary spherocytosis (HS) is also due to an underlying RBC membrane defect. The membrane defect in HS is in many instances due to spectrin, ankyrin, band 3 protein, or protein 4.2. The MCHC value may be increased in patients with HS.

◊ Schistocyte: Fragmented RBC

SCHISTOCYTE: FRAGMENTED RBC

Different variants can be seen
(helmet cell shown below)

Usually lacks
central pallor

|————————|10µm

Rashidi H MD, Nguyen J MD et al. HematologyOutlines.com

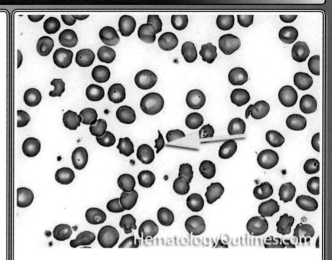

The arrow points at the fragmented RBC (schistocyte)

🔬 Microscopic Features
- Usually smaller than a normal RBC
- *Different RBC fragment variants (helmet cell, irregular fragments, etc.)*
- Usually lacks a central pallor

⚠ Frequency in Tissues
- Peripheral Blood: ○ Rare to ⊘ None
- Bone Marrow: ○ Rare to ⊘ None
- Lymph Node: ○ Rare to ⊘ None

↔ May Resemble
- Bite Cell {p. 97}
- Sickle Cell {p. 103}
- Spur cell (see in Glossary)
- Normal Mature RBC {p. 91}

ᴅx Differential Diagnoses
- ↑ Increased in:
  - Microangiopathic hemolytic anemia (e.g. as seen in DIC, TTP, or HUS)
  - Severe burns
  - Mechanical valve-induced
  - Uremia
  - Malignant hypertension

⚙ Classic Immunophenotype
- N/A

Miscellaneous: Usually associated with an intravascular hemolytic process (as opposed to spherocytes which are usually associated with an extravascular hemolytic process). In intravascular hemolytic conditions, haptoglobin levels are typically decreased.

◊ Schistocyte: Fragmented RBC

⬤ Stomatocyte

STOMATOCYTE

Same size as normal RBC

"Slit-like" or "Mouth-like"
central pallor

■——————■10µm

Rashidi H MD, Nguyen J MD et al. HematologyOutlines.com

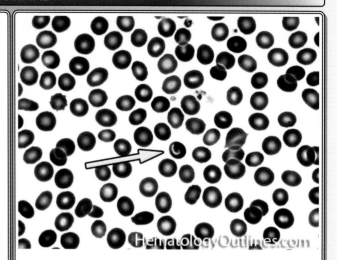

The arrow points at the mouth-shaped RBC.

🔬 Microscopic Features
- About the same size as a normal RBC
- *Slit-like or mouth-like central pallor (hence the term "stoma")*

⚠ Frequency in Tissues
- Peripheral Blood: ○ Rare to ⊘ None
- Bone Marrow: ○ Rare to ⊘ None
- Lymph Node: ○ Rare to ⊘ None

↔ May Resemble
- Normal Mature RBC {p. 91}
- Macrocytic RBC {p. 95}

Dx Differential Diagnoses
- Hereditary stomatocytosis
- Liver disease
- Tangier disease
- Rh null disease
- Artifact

⚙ Classic Immunophenotype
- N/A

Miscellaneous: Similar to hereditary spherocytosis, hereditary stomatocytosis is also due to an underlying RBC membrane defect.

◊ Target Cell RBC

TARGET CELL RBC

Normochromic to slightly macrocytic

Central dark region →

"Bull's eye" appearance

━━━━━━━10μm

Rashidi H MD, Nguyen J MD et al. HematologyOutlines.com

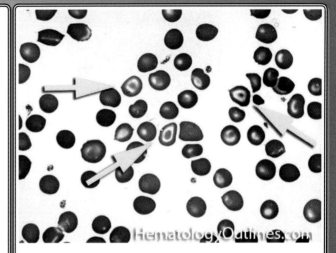

The arrows point to the target cells.

🔬 Microscopic Features
- About the same size as a normal RBC
- Round shape
- *Bullseye appearance (resembles a target sign)*

⚠ Frequency in Tissues
- Peripheral Blood: ○ Rare to ⊘ None
- Bone Marrow: ○ Rare to ⊘ None
- Lymph Node: ○ Rare to ⊘ None

↔ May Resemble
- Normal Mature RBC {p. 91}
- Macrocytic RBC {p. 95}
- Hemoglobin C Crystals {p. 105}

Dx Differential Diagnoses
- Thalassemia
- Hemoglobinopathies (C, SC, or E disease)
- Post-splenectomy
- Liver disease
- Artifact of slow drying of blood smear
- Iron deficiency anemia (sometimes)

⚙ Classic Immunophenotype
- N/A

Miscellaneous: Increased surface membrane to volume ratio gives rise to a central darker hemoglobinized region within the area of central pallor.

SICKLE CELL

Resembles a crescent or banana

Dense hemoglobin
No central pallor

━━━━━━━━10µm

Rashidi H MD, Nguyen J MD et al. HematologyOutlines.com

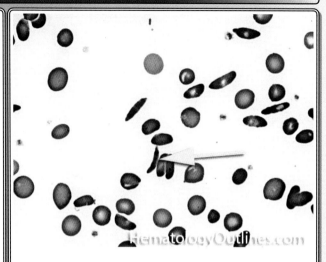

Multiple sickle cells are seen in this smear.

🔬 Microscopic Features
- About the same size as a normal RBC
- *Banana-shaped RBC with two pointed ends*
- Usually forming the shape of a crescent or banana
- Dense hemoglobin (dark red to light purple)
- No central pallor

⚠ Frequency in Tissues
- Peripheral Blood: ⊘ None
- Bone Marrow: ⊘ None
- Lymph Node: ⊘ None

↔ May Resemble
- Schistocyte {p. 100}
- Ovalocyte (elliptocyte) {p. 98}
- Hemoglobin C Crystals {p. 105}
- Malaria organisms (gametes outside of RBCs)

Dx Differential Diagnoses
- Hemoglobin SS disease
- Hemoglobin SC disease
- Hemoglobin SD disease
- S-beta thalassemia

⚙ Classic Immunophenotype
- N/A

Miscellaneous: Sickle cell disease arises from an underlying mutation in the hemoglobin beta chain. The hydrophilic amino acid residue glutamate is replaced with the hydrophobic amino acid residue valine, which leads to aggregation of the hemoglobin molecules that ultimately twists the RBC into a sickled shaped cell.

♦ Teardrop Cell

TEARDROP RBC

Unipolar tapered end
with a blunt tip

Teardrop or pear-shaped

■——————10µm

Rashidi H MD, Nguyen J MD et al. HematologyOutlines.com

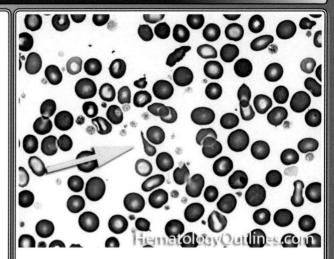

The arrow points at the tear-drop shaped RBC

🔬 Microscopic Features
- About the same size as a normal RBC
- The *RBC is teardrop or pear-shaped*

⚠ Frequency in Tissues
- Peripheral Blood: ⊘ None
- Bone Marrow: ⊘ None
- Lymph Node: ⊘ None

↔ May Resemble
- Normal Mature RBC {p. 91}
- Ovalocyte (elliptocyte) {p. 98}
- Schistocyte {p. 100}
- Sickle Cell {p. 103}

Dx Differential Diagnoses
- Myelofibrosis
- Bone marrow infiltration by hematologic or non-hematologic malignancy
- Artifact of slide preparation (in which all the tails usually point in the same direction)

⚙ Classic Immunophenotype
- N/A

Miscellaneous: Increased number of teardrop RBCs is a clue to a possible underlying marrow process (e.g. fibrosis, metastases).

Hemoglobin C Crystals

HEMOGLOBIN C CRYSTALS IN RBCS

Variable size of dense,
crystalline structures

10μm

Rashidi H MD, Nguyen J MD et al. HematologyOutlines.com

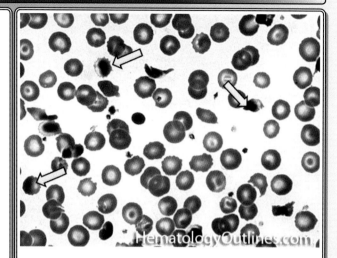

The arrows are highlighting the dark hemoglobin C
crystal inclusions.

🔬 Microscopic Features
- Variable sized RBC crystalline dark blue-purple inclusions
- *Hexagon-shaped or rhomboid shaped crystalline structures in RBCs*

⚠ Frequency in Tissues
- Peripheral Blood: ⊘ None
- Bone Marrow: ⊘ None
- Lymph Node: ⊘ None

↔ May Resemble
- Sickle Cell {p. 103}
- Bite Cell {p. 97}
- Target Cell {p. 102}

Dx Differential Diagnoses
- Hemoglobin C disease
- Hemoglobin SC disease

⚙ Classic Immunophenotype
- N/A

Miscellaneous: Hemoglobin C and SC patients may also show increased number of target cells.

🔴 Red Cell Agglutinate

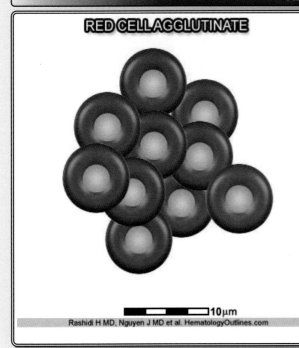

RED CELL AGGLUTINATE

10µm

Rashidi H MD, Nguyen J MD et al. HematologyOutlines.com

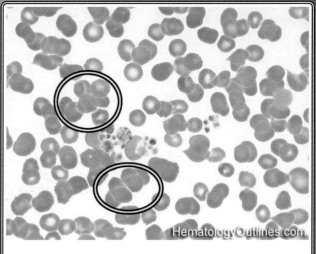

HematologyOutlines.com

The agglutinated RBCs are highlighted by the circles.

🔬 Microscopic Features

- Irregular overlapping aggregate of RBCs
- *A cluster of overlapping RBCs (non-linear overlapping RBCs)*

⚠️ Frequency in Tissues

- Peripheral Blood: ⊘ None
- Bone Marrow: ⊘ None
- Lymph Node: ⊘ None

↔️ May Resemble

- Rouleaux {p. 107}
- Thick area of a blood smear giving rise to overlapping RBCs

℞ Differential Diagnoses

- Paroxysmal cold hemoglobinuria
- Cold agglutinins
- Elevated serum IgM M-spike as in Waldenstrom's macroglobulinemia
- Plasma cell neoplasm associated with monoclonal IgM

⚙️ Classic Immunophenotype

- N/A

Miscellaneous: This finding must be evaluated in the appropriate section of the peripheral blood smear (where RBCs are usually not touching each other). Typically associated with cold antibodies (usually IgM). Mostly due to reduced zeta potential and van der Waals forces.

📝 **Note**: The zeta potential between RBCs keeps them apart. Hence anything that reduces this zeta potential (usually relatively positively charged molecules such as immunoglobulins) will facilitate RBCs to aggregate or stack on top of each other. Please see the zeta potential entry in the Glossary for more information.

🩸 Rouleaux

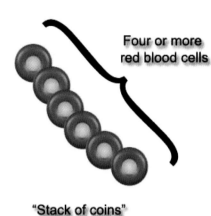

ROULEAUX

Four or more red blood cells

"Stack of coins" appearance

Rashidi H MD, Nguyen J MD et al. HematologyOutlines.com

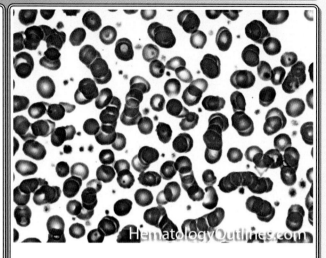

Rouleaux RBCs resemble "stack of coins"

🔬 Microscopic Features
- Stacking of four or more RBCs in a linear fashion
- *"Stack of coins" appearance*
- Must be in the correct location of the slide for definitive finding (slightly inside of the feathered edge)

⚠ Frequency in Tissues
- Peripheral Blood: ⊘ None
- Bone Marrow: ⊘ None
- Lymph Node: ⊘ None

↔ May Resemble
- Red Blood Cell Agglutinate {p. 106}
- Thick area of a blood smear may give rise to overlapping RBCs (Pseudo-Rouleaux)

Dx Differential Diagnoses
- Plasma cell neoplasms (e.g. plasma cell myeloma)
- Chronic liver disease with hypergammaglobulinemia
- Chronic infections
- Chronic inflammation
- Evaluating the wrong area of a slide (e.g. thick area of a blood smear with pseudo-rouleaux)

⚙ Classic Immunophenotype
- N/A

Miscellaneous: This finding must be evaluated in the appropriate section of the peripheral blood smear (where RBCs are usually not touching each other). Mostly due to reduced zeta potential.

Note: The zeta potential between RBCs keeps them apart. Hence anything that reduces this zeta potential (usually relatively positively charged molecules such as immunoglobulins) will facilitate RBCs to aggregate or stack on top of each other. Please see the zeta potential entry in the Glossary for more information.

Diagram of Red blood Cell Inclusions

Common RBC Inclusions	Cartoon Image	Inclusion	May be associated with
Howell Jolly Bodies		DNA	Hyposplenism Asplenism Severe hemolytic anemia
Heinz Bodies	*Supravital stain*	Hemoglobin	G6PD deficiency Oxidant drugs Unstable hemoglobin
Pappenheimer Bodies		Iron deposits	Thalassemia Sideroblastic anemia Hemolytic anemia Post-splenectomy
Hemoglobin H Inclusion	*Supravital stain*	Hemoglobin	Hemoglobin H disease
Basophilic Stippling		Ribosomes	Lead poisoning Thalassemia Sickle cell anemia MDS

Rashidi H MD, Yee N, Nguyen J MD et al. HematologyOutlines.com

Many different types of inclusions can be seen in RBCs and some may resemble microorganisms and even platelets.

HOWELL-JOLLY BODY

Spherical, dark
cytoplasmic inclusion

Iron stain negative
DNA stain positive

━━━━━━━━10μm

Rashidi H MD, Nguyen J MD et al. HematologyOutlines.com

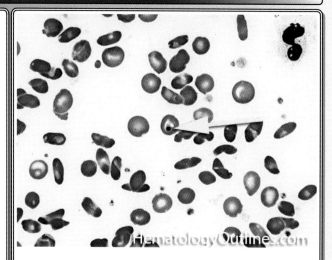

The arrow points at the RBC with a Howell-Jolly body

🔬 Microscopic Features
- ***Smooth round dark blue-purple cytoplasmic inclusion***
- May be centrally located or sometimes in the periphery
- Composed of fragments of DNA
- Iron stain negative

⚠️ Frequency in Tissues
- Peripheral Blood: ⊘ None
- Bone Marrow: ⊘ None
- Lymph Node: ⊘ None

↔ May Resemble
- Pappenheimer Bodies {p. 111}
- Basophilic Stippling {p. 113}
- Heinz Body {p. 110} (visible only with supravital stain)
- Hemoglobin H Inclusions {p. 112} (visible only with supravital stain)
- Malaria Infection {p. 115}
- Babesia Infection {p. 116}
- Fungal Infection {p. 121}
- Artifacts (e.g. Stain precipitate)

🅳ₓ Differential Diagnoses
- Asplenism (no spleen as in post-splenectomy)
- Severe hemolytic anemia (sometimes)

⚙️ Classic Immunophenotype
- N/A

Miscellaneous: Basophilic stippling is due to ribosomal inclusions in RBCs, while Pappenheimer bodies are from iron deposits, Heinz bodies are precipitated hemoglobin seen with special stain ("He" for Heinz and "He" for Hemoglobin), and Howell-Jolly bodies are from DNA remnants.

⬧ Heinz Bodies

HEINZ BODY

Purple-blue inclusions
visible only after supravital stains

Supravital stain:

Composed of denatured,
precipitated hemoglobin

▬▬▬▬▬▬10µm

Rashidi H MD, Nguyen J MD et al. HematologyOutlines.com

HematologyOutlines.com

Heinz bodies are not seen on routine stains. They are only seen with supravital stain.

🔬 Microscopic Features
- *Purple-blue inclusions visible only after supravital stain*
- Composed of denatures hemoglobin (usually oxidized hemoglobin)

⚠ Frequency in Tissues
- Peripheral Blood: ⊘ None
- Bone Marrow: ⊘ None
- Lymph Node: ⊘ None

↔ May Resemble
- Hemoglobin H Inclusions {p. 112} (visible only with supravital stain)
- Pappenheimer Bodies {p. 111} (visible with and without iron stain)
- Basophilic Stippling {p. 113}
- Howell-Jolly Body {p. 109}
- Malaria Infection {p. 115}
- Babesia Infection {p. 116}
- Fungal Infection {p. 121}
- Artifacts (e.g. stain precipitate)

Dx Differential Diagnoses
- G6PD deficiency
- Chemical poisoning-induced
- Oxidant drug-induced

⚙ Classic Immunophenotype
- N/A

Miscellaneous: Basophilic stippling is due to ribosomal inclusions in RBCs, while Pappenheimer bodies are from iron deposits, Heinz bodies are precipitated hemoglobin seen with special stain ("He" for Heinz and "He" for Hemoglobin), and Howell-Jolly bodies are from DNA remnants.

◊ Pappenheimer Bodies

PAPPENHEIMER BODY

Irregular, dark, blue-purple
granule(s) at periphery

Iron stain positive

━━━━━10μm

Rashidi H MD, Nguyen J MD et al. HematologyOutlines.com

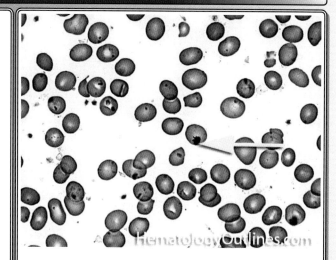

The arrow points to the Pappenheimer body in the RBC

🔬 Microscopic Features
- *Irregular, small blue-purple granular aggregates in RBCs*
- The granules are usually located at the periphery of the RBC

⚠ Frequency in Tissues
- Peripheral Blood: ⊘ None
- Bone Marrow: ⊘ None
- Lymph Node: ⊘ None

↔ May Resemble
- Howell-Jolly Body {p. 109} (iron stain negative)
- Basophilic Stippling {p. 113} (iron stain negative)
- Heinz Body {p. 110} (iron stain negative, visible only with supravital stain)
- Hemoglobin H Inclusions {p. 112} (iron stain negative, visible only with supravital stain)
- Malaria Infection {p. 115}
- Babesia Infection {p. 116}
- Fungal Infection {p. 121}
- Artifacts (e.g. stain precipitate)

Dx Differential Diagnoses
- Thalassemia
- Sideroblastic anemia
- Hemolytic anemia
- Post-splenenctomy

⚙ Classic Immunophenotype
- N/A

Miscellaneous: Basophilic stippling is due to ribosomal inclusions in RBCs, while Pappenheimer bodies are from iron deposits, Heinz bodies are precipitated hemoglobin seen with special stain ("He" for Heinz and "He" for Hemoglobin), and Howell-Jolly bodies are from DNA remnants. The aggregates are partially composed of iron but visible with and without iron stain (as opposed to a sideroblast's iron granules which are only visible with iron stain).

🔹 Hemoglobin H Inclusion

HEMOGLOBIN H INCLUSIONS

Many purple-blue inclusions
seen with supravital stain

Supravital stain:

Composed of precipitated
chains of beta-hemoglobin
(beta4 tetramers)

▭▭▭10µm

Rashidi H MD, Nguyen J MD et al. HematologyOutlines.com

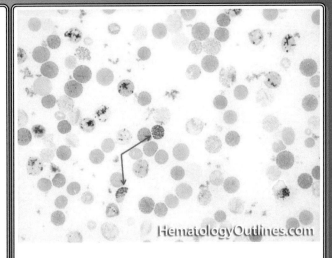

Requires supravital stain for visualization

🔬 Microscopic Features
- *Multiple small blue-purple granules distributed within an RBC and visualized with special stain*
- Composed of precipitated chains of beta-hemoglobin (tetramer of beta chains) seen in some alpha thalassemias

⚠ Frequency in Tissues
- Peripheral Blood: ⊘ None
- Bone Marrow: ⊘ None
- Lymph Node: ⊘ None

↔ May Resemble
- Heinz Bodies {p. 110} (visible only with supravital stain)
- Pappenheimer Bodies {p. 111}
- Howell-Jolly Body {p. 109}
- Basophilic Stippling {p. 113}
- Malaria Infection {p. 115}
- Babesia Infection {p. 116}
- Artifacts (e.g. stain precipitate)

ᴰˣ Differential Diagnoses
- Alpha thalassemia
- Myeloproliferative syndromes: sometimes
- Erythroleukemia (AML-M6): sometimes

⚙ Classic Immunophenotype
- N/A

Miscellaneous: These inclusions are seen with special supravital stain. In some alpha thalassemias, the decreased production of alpha chains leads to an excess of beta chains which can form beta-tetramers and precipitate.

ABNORMAL

BASOPHILIC STIPPLING

Variable size of granules
distributed throughout

Seen on Wright-Giemsa staining

━━━━━━━10μm

Rashidi H MD, Nguyen J MD et al. HematologyOutlines.com

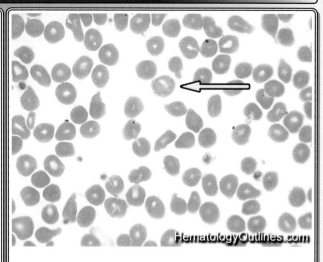

HematologyOutlines.com

The arrow points to the RBC with basophilic stippling

🔬 Microscopic Features
- *Very small (dot-like) blue or blue-gray granules distributed throughout the cytoplasm of RBCs*
- Composed of ribosomes

⚠ Frequency in Tissues
- Peripheral Blood: ⊘ None
- Bone Marrow: ⊘ None
- Lymph Node: ⊘ None

↔ May Resemble
- Pappenheimer Bodies {p. 111}
- Heinz Bodies {p. 110} (seen with supravital stain only)
- Howell-Jolly Body {p. 109}
- Hemoglobin H Inclusion {p. 112} (seen with supravital stain only)
- Malaria Infection {p. 115}
- Babesia Infection {p. 116}
- Giant Platelets {p. 155}
- Artifacts (e.g. stain precipitate)

Dx Differential Diagnoses
- Lead poisoning
- Thalassemia
- Sickle cell anemia
- Myelodysplastic syndrome (MDS)

⚙ Classic Immunophenotype
- N/A

Miscellaneous: Basophilic stippling is due to ribosomal inclusions in RBCs, while Pappenheimer bodies are from iron deposits, Heinz bodies are precipitated hemoglobin seen with special stain ("He" for Heinz and "He" for Hemoglobin), and Howell-Jolly bodies are from DNA remnants.

Infections Involving Peripheral Blood

Microorganisms in Blood	Cartoon Image	Features
Malaria	*Trophozoite* *Schizont*	**Multiple states of organism development seen in peripheral blood**
Babesia		**Distinguished from malaria by tetrad arrangement of merozoites**
Trypanosoma		**Extracellular parasite**
Microfilaria		**Very large parasite (Compared to Malaria, Babesia, or Trypanosoma)**
Bacterial contamination in peripheral blood smear		**Usually from contamination of blood film by skin flora**
Borrelia		**Very thin spiral shaped extracellular bacteria**
Candida		**Usually smaller than the surrounding RBCs** **Occasional budding may be noted**

Rashidi H MD, Yee N, Nguyen J MD et al. HematologyOutlines.com

These are a sample of infectious agents that can be found in peripheral blood.

🩸 Infectious-Malaria

RBCs : INFECTIOUS - MALARIA

Example of trophozoite

Example of schizont

10μm

Rashidi H MD, Nguyen J MD et al. HematologyOutlines.com

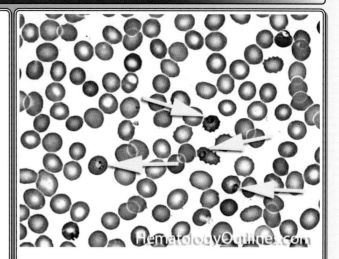

The arrows point at the malaria organisms in the RBCs

🔬 Microscopic Features
- *Infects RBCs*
- Round to oval ring-shaped intracellular parasite in RBCs
- Usually <2 μm in young trophozoites
- Later stage trophozoites may be as big as a RBC (4-8 μm)
- Schizonts & gametocytes may be even larger than RBCs (5-10 μm)
- Gametocyte forms are banana shaped and usually associated with falciparum species

⚠ Frequency in Tissues
- Peripheral Blood: ⊘ None
- Bone Marrow: ⊘ None
- Lymph Node: ⊘ None

↔ May Resemble
- Babesia Infection {p. 116}
- Platelet overlying red blood cell
- Howell-Jolly Body {p. 109}
- Pappenheimer Bodies {p. 111}
- Bacterial Contamination {p. 119}
- Artifacts (e.g. stain precipitate)

Dx Differential Diagnoses
- Babesia
- Platelet overlying a RBC (pseudo-parasite)

⚙ Classic Immunophenotype
- N/A

Miscellaneous: Malarial infection is predominantly an intracellular parasite (infects RBCs). The extracellular banana-shaped gametocyte is usually associated with the falciparum species (clinically very significant).

Infectious-Babesia

RBCs: INFECTIOUS - BABESIA

"Maltese cross"
merozoite form

━━━━━━━ 10μm

Rashidi H MD, Nguyen J MD et al. HematologyOutlines.com

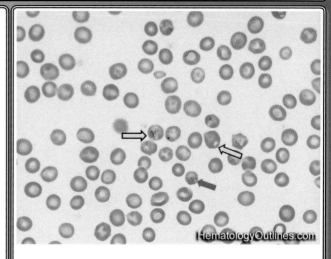

The red arrows point to the "Maltese cross." The yellow arrows point to the organisms.

Microscopic Features
- *Multiple parasites may be present within an RBC*
- Round to oval ring-shaped and mostly intracellular parasites in RBCs
- The organisms may form a "Maltese cross" after division into four organisms

Frequency in Tissues
- Peripheral Blood: ⊘ None
- Bone Marrow: ⊘ None
- Lymph Node: ⊘ None

May Resemble
- Malaria Infection {p. 115}
- Howell-Jolly Body {p. 109}
- Pappenheimer Bodies {p. 111}
- Bacterial Contamination {p. 119}
- Platelet(s) overlying red blood cell
- Artifacts (e.g. stain precipitate)

Differential Diagnoses
- Malaria
- Platelet overlying a RBC (pseudo-parasite)

Classic Immunophenotype
- N/A

Miscellaneous: Distinguished from malaria by having a tetrad arrangement which is usually diagnostic of babesia. It is also an intracellular parasite (infects RBCs).

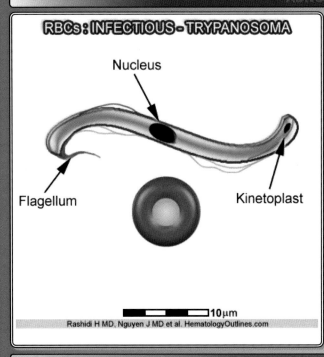

RBCs : INFECTIOUS - TRYPANOSOMA

Nucleus

Flagellum

Kinetoplast

10µm

Rashidi H MD, Nguyen J MD et al. HematologyOutlines.com

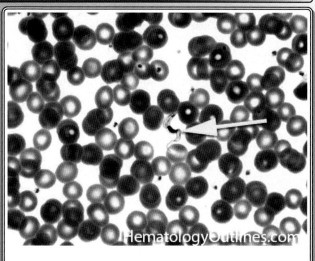

HematologyOutlines.com

The arrow points to the parasite, which is slightly larger than the size of a red blood cell.

🔬 Microscopic Features
- *Swirl-shaped (worm shaped) extracellular parasite*
- The length is twice that of the RBC diameter and the width is ~1/2-1/3 that of a RBC diameter

⚠️ Frequency in Tissues
- Peripheral Blood: ⊘ None
- Bone Marrow: ⊘ None
- Lymph Node: ⊘ None

↔️ May Resemble
- Microfilaria {p. 118}
- Malaria Infection {p. 115}
- Sickle Cell {p. 103}

Dx Differential Diagnoses
- Other parasites
- Artifact

⚙️ Classic Immunophenotype
- N/A

Miscellaneous: This is an extracellular parasite.

⬥ Infectious-Microfilaria

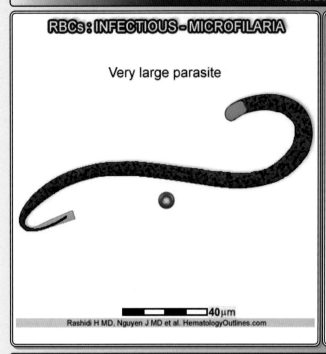

RBCs : INFECTIOUS – MICROFILARIA

Very large parasite

|40 μm

Rashidi H MD, Nguyen J MD et al. HematologyOutlines.com

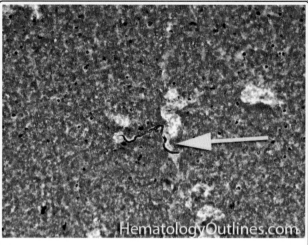

The arrow points to the very large parasite at low power.

🔬 Microscopic Features
- *Very large parasites (as compared to other parasites such as malaria, babesia, or even Trypanosoma)*
- Worm-like appearance
- Extracellular parasites

⚠ Frequency in Tissues
- Peripheral Blood: ⊘ None
- Bone Marrow: ⊘ None
- Lymph Node: ⊘ None

↔ May Resemble
- Trypanosoma {p. 117}

ᴰx Differential Diagnoses
- Other parasites
- Artifact (cloth, etc.)

⚙ Classic Immunophenotype
- N/A

Miscellaneous: This is an extracellular parasite. One must scan the peripheral blood smear on very low power first to make sure it is not missed.

Bacterial contamination in peripheral blood

BACTERIAL CONTAMINATION RBCS

Usually cocci in chains

|—————————|10µm

Rashidi H MD, Nguyen J MD et al. HematologyOutlines.com

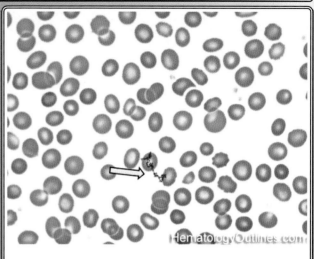

The arrow points to the clusters of bacterial cocci (likely contaminant)

⚕ Microscopic Features
- *Bacterial colonies (usually cocci in chains and clusters) over RBCs*
- The contaminating bacteria are usually cocci (dark blue round structures much smaller than the RBC)

⚠ Frequency in Tissues
- Peripheral Blood: ⊘ None
- Bone Marrow: ⊘ None
- Lymph Node: ⊘ None

↔ May Resemble
- Platelets overlying red blood cell
- Artifacts (e.g. stain precipitate)
- Real bacterial infection

℞x Differential Diagnoses
- Artifact
- Real bacterial infection involving blood

☼ Classic Immunophenotype
- N/A

Miscellaneous: Bacterial colonies, usually cocci (most likely Staphlococcus epidermidis), from contaminated handling during the processing of the peripheral blood smear by the medical technologist.

⬧ Infectious-Borrelia

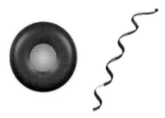

BORRELIA

Thin spiral-shaped
extracellular bacteria

━━━━━━━━━10μm

Rashidi H MD, Nguyen J MD et al. HematologyOutlines.com

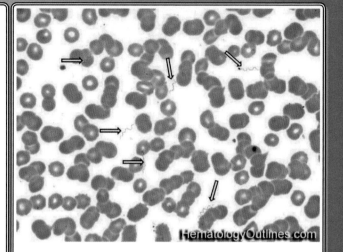

The arrows point to the spirochetes

🔬 Microscopic Features
- *Very thin spiral shaped extracellular bacteria known as a spirochete*

⚠ Frequency in Tissues
- Peripheral Blood: ⊘ None
- Bone Marrow: ⊘ None
- Lymph Node: ⊘ None

↔ May Resemble
- Trypanosoma {p. 117}
- Microfilaria {p. 118}
- Malaria Infection {p. 115}
- Sickle Cell {p. 103}

Ðx Differential Diagnoses
- Bacterial infection
- Parasitic infection
- Artifact

⚙ Classic Immunophenotype
- N/A

Miscellaneous: A spirochete that causes borreliosis (a disease typically transmitted by ticks). Multiple species exist including Borrelia burgdorferi which causes Lyme disease.

🩸 Infectious-Fungus (Candida)

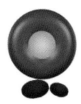

CANDIDA

Occasional budding
may be noted

Many have a
round-to-oval shape

⬛━━━━━□━━□10μm

Rashidi H MD, Nguyen J MD et al. HematologyOutlines.com

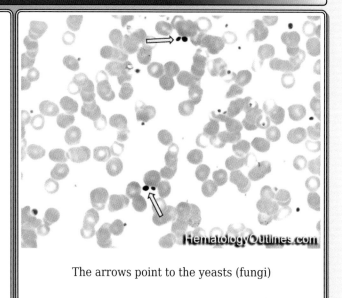

The arrows point to the yeasts (fungi)

🔬 Microscopic Features
- *Usually smaller than the surrounding RBCs*
- Many have a round to oval shape
- Occasional budding may be noted

⚠ Frequency in Tissues
- Peripheral Blood: ⊘ None
- Bone Marrow: ⊘ None
- Lymph Node: ⊘ None

↔ May Resemble
- Babesia Infection {p. 116}
- Malaria Infection {p. 115}
- Platelets {p. 153}
- Howell-Jolly Body {p. 109}
- Pappenheimer Bodies {p. 111}
- Bacterial Contamination {p. 119}
- Artifacts (e.g. stain precipitate)

Dx Differential Diagnoses
- Fungal infection
- Fungal contamination
- Malaria
- Babesia
- Artifact: Platelet overlying a RBC (pseudo-fungus)

✿ Classic Immunophenotype
- N/A

Miscellaneous: Fungi can present in the form of a yeast, hyphae, or both yeast and hyphae. Candidia is usually a yeast form with occasional pseudo-hyphae.

Granulocytic Maturation Overview Diagram

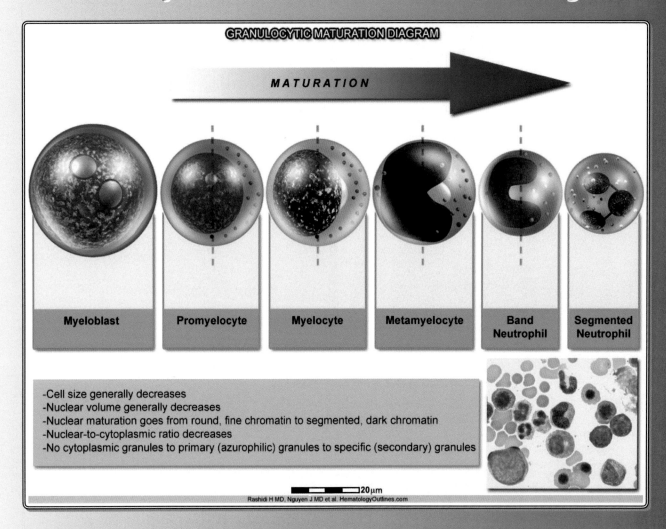

GRANULOCYTIC MATURATION DIAGRAM

MATURATION

| Myeloblast | Promyelocyte | Myelocyte | Metamyelocyte | Band Neutrophil | Segmented Neutrophil |

-Cell size generally decreases
-Nuclear volume generally decreases
-Nuclear maturation goes from round, fine chromatin to segmented, dark chromatin
-Nuclear-to-cytoplasmic ratio decreases
-No cytoplasmic granules to primary (azurophilic) granules to specific (secondary) granules

20 μm

Rashidi H MD, Nguyen J MD et al. HematologyOutlines.com

The overall trend in the series is from larger to smaller size; round, fine nucleus to dark, segmented nucleus; increasing cytoplasm; no granules to primary (azurophilic) granules to specific (secondary) granules.

💧 Myeloblast

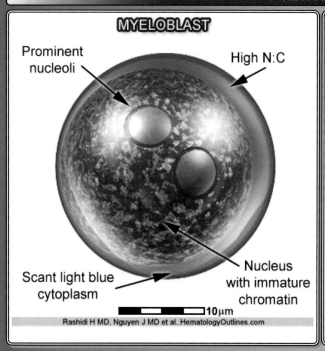

MYELOBLAST

Prominent nucleoli

High N:C

Scant light blue cytoplasm

Nucleus with immature chromatin

10µm

Rashidi H MD, Nguyen J MD et al. HematologyOutlines.com

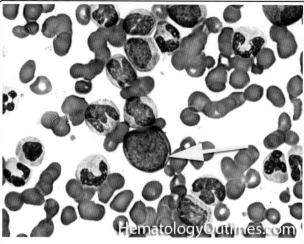

The yellow arrow points to a myeloblast. Notice the high N:C ratio, prominent nucleoli, and open chromatin.

🔬 Microscopic Features

- 3-4X larger than a mature RBC
- *High nuclear-to-cytoplasmic ratio*
- Round nucleus with immature chromatin (not clumped)
- Prominent nucleoli
- Cytoplasm is scant, gray to pale blue and lacks granules

⚠ Frequency in Tissues

- Peripheral Blood: ⊘ None
- Bone Marrow: 1-3%
- Lymph Node: ⊘ None

↔ May Resemble

- Promyelocyte {p. 22}
- Pronormoblast {p. 9}
- Lymphoblasts {p. 65}
- Immature B-cell (hematogone) {p. 62}
- Monoblast {p. 38}
- Reactive Lymphocyte {p. 137}

Dx Differential Diagnoses

- Acute myeloid leukemia (AML)
- Myelodysplastic syndromes (e.g. RAEB-I or II)
- Myeloproliferative neoplasms (e.g. CML with increased blasts)
- Leukemoid reactions
- Post GCSF therapy

⚙ Classic Immunophenotype

- CD34 ➕
- CD117 ➕
- HLA-DR ➕
- CD13 ➕
- CD33 **dim** ➕
- CD15 ➖
- MPO ➖/➕

Miscellaneous: A myeloblast with Auer rod(s) is by definition abnormal and usually represents an underlying AML or high grade MDS (MDS Excess Blasts 2 (MDS-EB-2) also known as Refractory Anemia with Excess Blasts 2 (RAEB-2)).

Promyelocyte

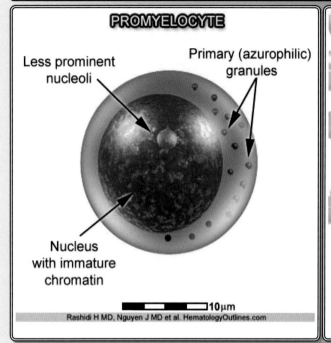

PROMYELOCYTE

Less prominent nucleoli

Primary (azurophilic) granules

Nucleus with immature chromatin

10μm

Rashidi H MD, Nguyen J MD et al. HematologyOutlines.com

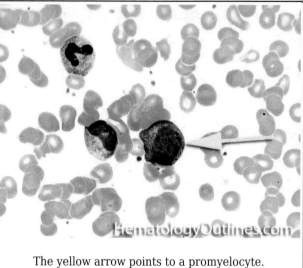

The yellow arrow points to a promyelocyte.

Microscopic Features
- 2-3X larger than a mature RBC
- *High nuclear-to-cytoplasmic ratio (but more cytoplasm than a myeloblast)*
- Round nucleus with immature chromatin (not clumped)
- Nucleoli are present but less prominent than myeloblasts
- Small amount of cytoplasm with primary (azurophilic) granules

Frequency in Tissues
- Peripheral Blood: ⊘ None
- Bone Marrow: 2-6%
- Lymph Node: ⊘ None

May Resemble
- Myeloblast {p. 21}
- Myelocyte {p. 23}
- Metamyelocyte {p. 24}
- Reactive Lymphocyte {p. 137}
- Neutrophil With Toxic Granules {p. 131}
- Segmented Neutrophil {p. 26}
- Large Granular Lymphocyte {p. 138}

Differential Diagnoses
- Acute promyelocytic leukemia (AML M3)
- Myeloproliferative neoplasms (e.g. CML)
- Leukemoid reactions
- Post GCSF therapy

Classic Immunophenotype
- CD34 ⊖
- CD117 ⊞
- HLA-DR ⊖
- CD13 ⊞
- CD33 ⊞
- CD15 ⊖ / ⊞
- MPO ⊞

Miscellaneous: This development stage is the maturation step that comes after myeloblast and precedes myelocyte.

🔹 Myelocyte

ABNORMAL

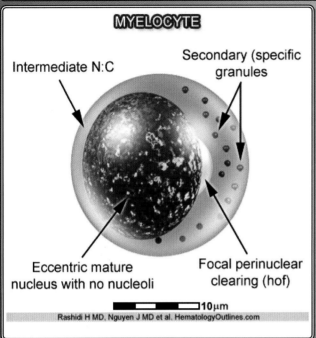

MYELOCYTE

Intermediate N:C

Secondary (specific) granules

Eccentric mature nucleus with no nucleoli

Focal perinuclear clearing (hof)

10μm

Rashidi H MD, Nguyen J MD et al. HematologyOutlines.com

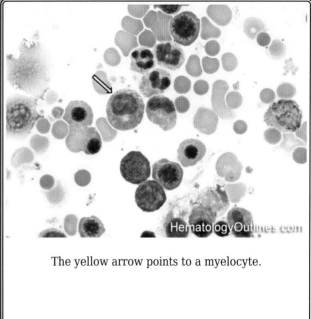

The yellow arrow points to a myelocyte.

🔬 Microscopic Features
- 2-3X larger than a mature RBC
- Intermediate nuclear-to-cytoplasmic ratio (more cytoplasm than promyelocyte)
- ***Eccentrically placed oval nucleus (no nucleus indentation) with more mature chromatin (clumped)***
- Perinuclear clearing is common
- Nucleoli are absent (Note: nucleoli are absent from this stage onward)
- More cytoplasm with only rare or absent primary (azurophilic) granules
- Secondary (specific) granules of neutrophilic (lilac), eosinophilic (red-orange), or basophilic (blue) color are present based on precursor type

⚠ Frequency in Tissues
- Peripheral Blood: ⊘ None
- Bone Marrow: ~10%
- Lymph Node: ⊘ None

↔ May Resemble
- Promyelocyte {p. 124}
- Metamyelocyte {p. 126}
- Monocyte {p. 144}
- Reactive Lymphocyte {p. 137}
- Plasma Cell {p. 67}

ᴅₓ Differential Diagnoses
- ↑ Increased in:
  - ○ Chronic myelogenous leukemia (CML)
  - ○ Leukemoid reaction
  - ○ Post GCSF therapy

⚙ Classic Immunophenotype
- CD34 ⊖, HLA-DR ⊖ and CD117 ⊖
- CD13 **dim** ⊞
- CD33 ⊞
- CD15 ⊞
- CD11b ⊞ / ⊖
- CD16 ⊖
- MPO ⊞

Miscellaneous: This is the maturation step that comes after promyelocyte and precedes metamyelocyte.

🩸 Metamyelocyte

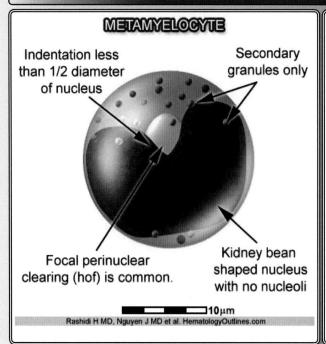

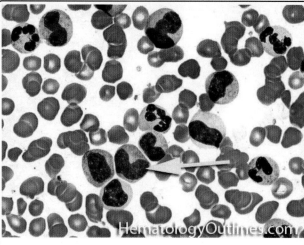

The yellow arrow points to a metamyelocyte. Note the nuclear indentation.

🔬 Microscopic Features

- 2-3X larger than a mature RBC
- Intermediate nuclear-to-cytoplasmic (N:C) ratio (more cytoplasm than a promyelocyte)
- *Kidney bean shaped nucleus (indent is less than 1/2 diameter) and mature chromatin (clumped)*
- Perinuclear clearing is common
- Nucleoli are absent
- More cytoplasm with only secondary granules
- Secondary (specific) granules of neutrophilic (lilac), eosinophilic (red-orange), or basophilic (blue) color are present based on precursor type

⚠ Frequency in Tissues

- Peripheral Blood: ⊘ None
- Bone Marrow: ~15%
- Lymph Node: ⊘ None

↔ May Resemble

- Promyelocyte {p. 22}
- Myelocyte {p. 23}
- Band Neutrophil {p. 25}
- Monocyte {p. 40}
- Reactive Lymphocyte {p. 137}
- Mature Segmented Neutrophil {p. 26}

ᴅx Differential Diagnoses

- ↑ Increased in:
  - Chronic myelogenous leukemia (CML)
  - Leukemoid reaction
  - Post GCSF therapy

⚙ Classic Immunophenotype

- CD34 ⊖, CD117 ⊖, and HLA-DR ⊖
- CD13 ⊞ and CD33 ⊞
- CD15 ⊞
- CD11b ⊞
- CD16 ⊞
- MPO ⊞

Miscellaneous: This is the maturation step that comes after myelocyte and precedes the band neutrophil.

◊ Band Neutrophil

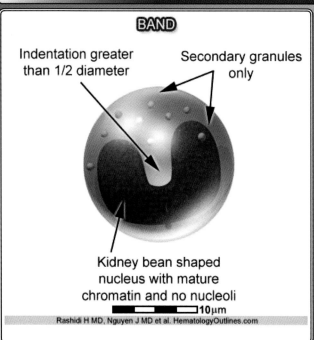

BAND

Indentation greater than 1/2 diameter

Secondary granules only

Kidney bean shaped nucleus with mature chromatin and no nucleoli

10μm

Rashidi H MD, Nguyen J MD et al. HematologyOutlines.com

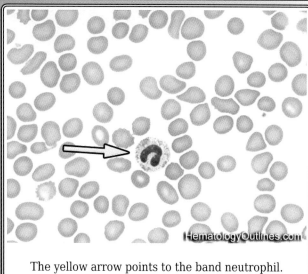

The yellow arrow points to the band neutrophil.

🔬 Microscopic Features

- 2-3X larger than a mature RBC
- Low nuclear-to-cytoplasmic (N:C) ratio (cytoplasm is relatively increased)
- *Kidney bean-shaped nucleus with indentation (>1/2 the diameter of the nucleus is indented) and mature chromatin (clumped)*
- Nucleoli are absent
- More cytoplasm with only secondary granules
- Secondary (specific) granules of neutrophilic (lilac), eosinophilic (red-orange), or basophilic (blue) color are present based on precursor type

⚠ Frequency in Tissues

- Peripheral Blood: ○ Rare (~1-5%)
- Bone Marrow: ✦ Scattered (~10-15%)
- Lymph Node: ○ Rare to ⊘ None

↔ May Resemble

- Segmented Neutrophil {p. 26}
- Metamyelocyte {p. 24}
- Myelocyte {p. 23}
- Promyelocyte {p. 22}
- Monocyte {p. 40}

Dx Differential Diagnoses

- Infections (especially bacterial)
- Myeloproliferative disorders (e.g. CML)
- Leukemoid reaction due to stress, etc.
- Post-GCSF therapy

⚙ Classic Immunophenotype

- CD34 ⊖, CD117 ⊖, and HLA-DR ⊖
- CD13 ⊕ and CD33 ⊕
- CD15 ⊕
- CD11b ⊕
- CD16 ⊕
- MPO ⊕
- CD10 ⊕ / ⊖

Miscellaneous: In normal blood, the band forms are almost all neutrophilic, while eosinophilic and basophilic band forms are confined to the bone marrow when present.

⬥ Segmented Neutrophil

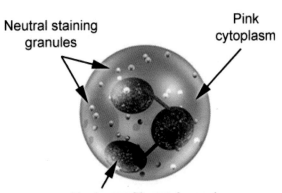

SEGMENTED NEUTROPHIL

Neutral staining granules

Pink cytoplasm

Nucleus with condensed clumped chromatin and 3 to 5 lobes connected by thin chromatin filaments

10μm

Rashidi H MD, Nguyen J MD et al. HematologyOutlines.com

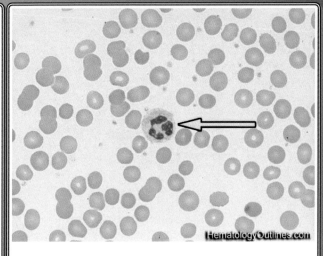

The yellow arrow points to the segmented neutrophil.

🔬 Microscopic Features
- 2-3X larger than a mature RBC
- Low nuclear-to-cytoplasmic ratio (more cytoplasm than nucleus)
- *Nucleus is mature and divided into 3 to 5 lobes connected by thin chromatin filaments*
- Nucleoli are absent
- More cytoplasm with only secondary granules
- Secondary (specific) granules are neutrophilic (lilac)

⚠ Frequency in Tissues
- Peripheral Blood: ⬤ Many (most common WBC)
- Bone Marrow: ⚙ Scattered
- Lymph Node: ○ Rare to ⊘ None

↔ May Resemble
- Hypersegmented Neutrophil {p. 130}
- Pseudo-Pelger Huet Neutrophil {p. 132}
- Band Neutrophil {p. 25}
- Neutrophil With Toxic Granules {p. 131}
- Metamyelocyte {p. 24}
- Myelocyte {p. 23}
- Promyelocyte {p. 22}
- Monocyte {p. 40}

ᴅx Differential Diagnoses
- Infections (especially bacterial infections)
- Myeloproliferative disorders (e.g. CML and CNL)
- Leukemoid reaction
- Drug-induced

⚙ Classic Immunophenotype
- CD34 ⊖, CD117 ⊖, and HLA-DR ⊖
- CD10 ⊞, CD13 ⊞ and CD33 ⊞
- CD15 ⊞
- CD11b ⊞
- CD16 ⊞
- MPO ⊞

Miscellaneous: Normal segmentation is 3-5 lobes while hypersegmentation is greater than 5 lobes and hyposegmentation is less than 3 lobes.

ABNORMAL

MAY-HEGGLIN ANOMALY

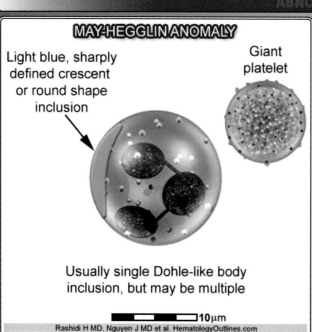

Light blue, sharply defined crescent or round shape inclusion

Giant platelet

Usually single Dohle-like body inclusion, but may be multiple

⊢━━━━━⊣10μm

Rashidi H MD, Nguyen J MD et al. HematologyOutlines.com

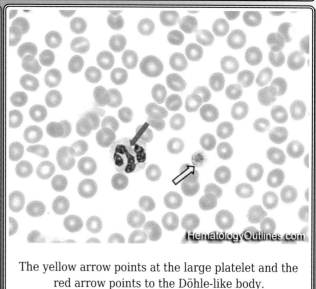

HematologyOutlines.com

The yellow arrow points at the large platelet and the red arrow points to the Döhle-like body.

🔬 Microscopic Features
- *Characterized by neutrophils with prominent Döhle-like bodies and background giant platelets*
- The Döhle-like bodies are half the diameter of an RBC with a light blue crescent shaped appearance
- Besides the neutrophils, other granulocytes, monocytes, and lymphocytes may also be involved

⚠ Frequency in Tissues
- Peripheral Blood: ⊘ None
- Bone Marrow: ⊘ None
- Lymph Node: ⊘ None

↔ May Resemble
- Chediak-Higashi Inclusions {p. 134}
- Neutrophil With Toxic Granules {p. 131}
- Segmented Neutrophil {p. 128}

Dx Differential Diagnoses
- Infection associated

⚙ Classic Immunophenotype
- N/A

Miscellaneous: May Hegglin anomaly usually demonstrates neutrophils with Döhle-like body inclusions and background giant platelets. Associated with mutation in MYH-9 (Myosin Heavy Chain gene).

⬧ Hypersegmented Neutrophil

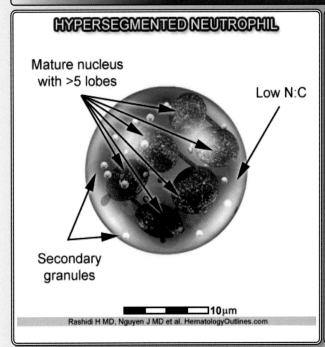

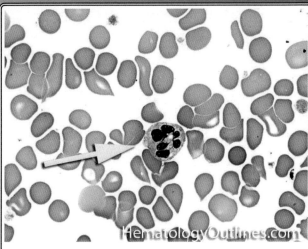

The arrow points to the hypersegmented neutrophil with 6 lobes.

🔬 Microscopic Features
- 3X larger than a mature RBC
- Low nuclear-to-cytoplasmic ratio (more cytoplasm than nucleus)
- *Nucleus is mature and has >5 lobes connected by thin chromatin filaments*
- Nucleoli are absent
- More cytoplasm with only secondary granules
- Secondary (specific) granules are neutrophilic (lilac)

⚠ Frequency in Tissues
- Peripheral Blood: ⊘ None
- Bone Marrow: ⊘ None
- Lymph Node: ⊘ None

↔ May Resemble
- Segmented Neutrophil {p. 128}
- Neutrophil With Toxic Granules {p. 131}
- Monocyte {p. 144}

ᴰx Differential Diagnoses
- Vitamin B12 deficiency
- Folate deficiency

⚙ Classic Immunophenotype
- CD45 ➕
- High SCC (side light scatter)
- CD10 ➕
- CD11b ➕
- CD13 ➕
- CD16 ➕

Miscellaneous: Usually associated with B12 or folate deficiency.

🔴 Neutrophil with Toxic Granules

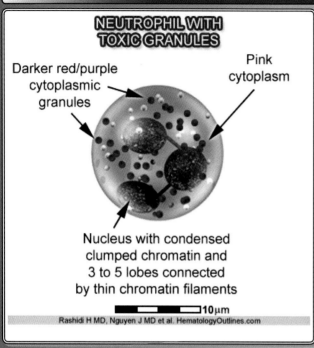

Darker red/purple cytoplasmic granules

Pink cytoplasm

Nucleus with condensed clumped chromatin and 3 to 5 lobes connected by thin chromatin filaments

10µm

Rashidi H MD, Nguyen J MD et al. HematologyOutlines.com

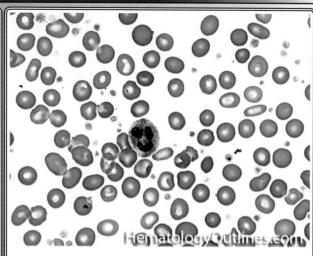

Note the darker staining granules compared to those seen in a normal neutrophil.

🔬 Microscopic Features
- 2-3X larger than a mature RBC
- Low nuclear-to-cytoplasmic ratio (more cytoplasm than nucleus)
- Nucleus is mature and divided into 3 to 5 lobes connected by thin chromatin filaments
- Nucleoli are absent
- *Darker (red/purple) granules are easily noted (similar to primary granules in promyelocytes)*

⚠ Frequency in Tissues
- Peripheral Blood: ○ Rare to ⊘ None
- Bone Marrow: ○ Rare to ⊘ None
- Lymph Node: ⊘ None

↔ May Resemble
- Segmented Neutrophil {p. 128}
- Hypersegmented Neutrophil {p. 130}
- Pseudo-Pelger Huet Neutrophil {p. 132}
- Band Neutrophil {p. 127}
- Large Granular Lymphocyte {p. 138}
- Promyelocyte {p. 124}
- Monocyte {p. 144}

Dx Differential Diagnoses
- Infection
- Inflammatory conditions

⚙ Classic Immunophenotype
- CD45 ➕ with high SCC
- CD10 ➕
- CD11b ➕
- CD13 ➕
- CD16 ➕

Miscellaneous: Usually associated with an underlying infection or inflammation. Neutrophils in infectious processes may also show vacuoles in the cytoplasm.

⬤ Pseudo Pelger Huet Neutrophil

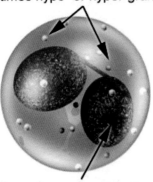

PSEUDO PELGER-HUET NEUTROPHIL

Lack of normal cytoplasmic granules
(sometimes hypo- or hyper-granulation)

Irregular nuclear lobation
(usually hypolobated)

10μm

Rashidi H MD, Nguyen J MD et al. HematologyOutlines.com

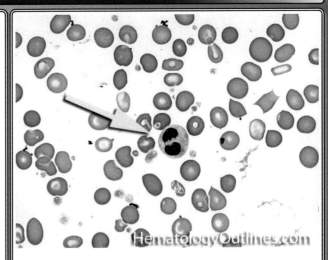

The yellow arrow points to the bilobed pseudo Pelger Huet neutrophil (2 lobes, instead of the normal 3-5 lobes)

🔬 Microscopic Features

- 2-3X larger than a mature RBC
- Low nuclear-to-cytoplasmic ratio (more cytoplasm than nucleus)
- *Nucleus is mature with 2 lobes connected by a thin chromatin filament*
- Nucleoli are absent
- In some cases, hypergranulation, hypogranulation or abnormal granules can be seen
- Pseudo Pelger-Huet neutrophils are a form of dysplastic neutrophils

⚠ Frequency in Tissues

- Peripheral Blood: ○ Rare to ⊘ None
- Bone Marrow: ○ Rare to ⊘ None
- Lymph Node: ⊘ None

↔ May Resemble

- Eosinophil {p. 148}
- Segmented Neutrophil {p. 128}
- Band Neutrophil {p. 127}
- Neutrophil With Toxic Granules {p. 131}
- Basophil {p. 151}

⏷x Differential Diagnoses

- Myelodysplastic syndrome (MDS)
- Pelger Huet anomaly (if they are true Pelger Huet cells)

⚙ Classic Immunophenotype

- CD45 ⊞
- Lowered SCC (side scatter)
- CD10 ⊟ / ⊞
- CD11b ⊞ / ⊟
- CD13 ⊞ / ⊟
- CD16 ⊞ / ⊟

Miscellaneous: Normal segmentation is 3-5 lobes while hyposegmentation is 5 lobes. The immunoprofile may be aberrant if it is dysplastic and associated with MDS.

⬥ Hypogranular or Agranular Neutrophil

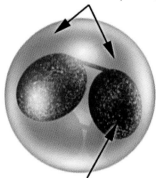

HYPOGRANULAR OR AGRANULAR NEUTROPHIL

Lack or diminished neutrophilic granules

Mature nucleus with two lobes
connected by thin chromatin filament

▬▬▬▬▬▬▬10μm

Rashidi H MD, Nguyen J MD et al. HematologyOutlines.com

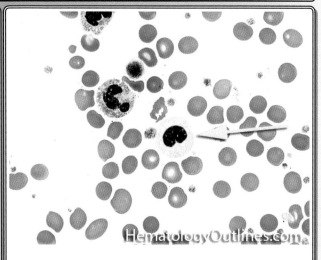

The yellow arrow points to the hypogranular (lack of granules) band neutrophil.

🔬 Microscopic Features
- 2-3X larger than a mature RBC
- Low nuclear-to-cytoplasmic ratio (more cytoplasm than nucleus)
- Nucleus is mature
- Nucleoli are absent
- *Lack or diminished neutrophilic granules*

⚠ Frequency in Tissues
- Peripheral Blood: ○ Rare to ⊘ None
- Bone Marrow: ○ Rare to ⊘ None
- Lymph Node: ⊘ None

↔ May Resemble
- Segmented Neutrophil {p. 26}
- Band Neutrophil {p. 25}
- Monocyte {p. 40}

Dx Differential Diagnoses
- Myelodysplastic syndrome (MDS)
- Staining artifact giving rise to pseudo-hypogranularity

⚙ Classic Immunophenotype
- CD45 ➕
- Lowered SCC
- CD10 ➕/➖
- CD11b ➕/➖
- CD13 ➕/➖
- CD16 ➕/➖

Miscellaneous: The low side scatter (SCC) noted on flow cytometry analysis is due to the hypogranularity. The immunoprofile may be aberrant if it is dysplastic and associated with MDS.

🔥 Chediak Higashi Neutrophils

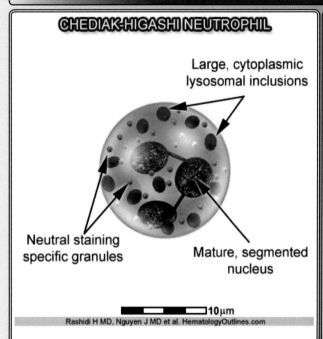

CHEDIAK-HIGASHI NEUTROPHIL

Large, cytoplasmic lysosomal inclusions

Neutral staining specific granules

Mature, segmented nucleus

10μm

Rashidi H MD, Nguyen J MD et al. HematologyOutlines.com

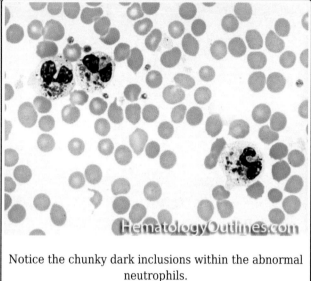

Notice the chunky dark inclusions within the abnormal neutrophils.

🔬 Microscopic Features
- Abnormal cytoplasmic inclusions invlolving the white blood cells (neutrophils, monocytes, eosinophils and lymphocytes)
- *Variably sized large aggregates of purple/blue/red granules*

⚠ Frequency in Tissues
- Peripheral Blood: ⊘ None
- Bone Marrow: ⊘ None
- Lymph Node: ⊘ None

↔ May Resemble
- Eosinophil {p. 148}
- Segmented Neutrophil {p. 128}
- Band Neutrophil {p. 127}
- Neutrophil With Toxic Granules {p. 131}
- Basophil {p. 151}

Dx Differential Diagnoses
- Chediak Higashi syndrome
- Infection
- Myelodysplastic syndrome (MDS)
- Inflammation

⚙ Classic Immunophenotype
- N/A

Miscellaneous: This disorder is due to the abnormal fusion of primary granules which results in a malfunctioning WBC with a diminished phagocytic capability. The syndrome is characterized by pancytopenia, neuropathy, oculocuteneous albinism, hepatosplenomegaly, lymphadenopathy, and recurrent infections.

⬥ Lymphocyte-Normal

NORMAL

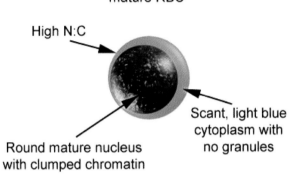

LYMPHOCYTE

Slightly larger than
mature RBC

High N:C

Round mature nucleus
with clumped chromatin

Scant, light blue
cytoplasm with
no granules

10µm

Rashidi H MD, Nguyen J MD et al. HematologyOutlines.com

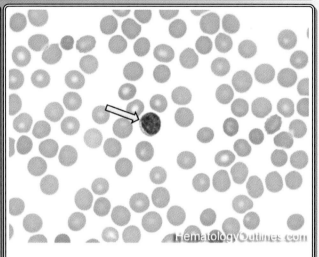

The nucleus is nearly the size of a mature RBC.

🔬 Microscopic Features
- ***Slightly (1.5X) larger than a mature RBC***
- High nuclear-to-cytoplasmic ratio but with a round mature nucleus (clumped chromatin)
- Nucleoli are absent
- Cytoplasm is scant, light blue and lacks granules

⚠ Frequency in Tissues
- Peripheral Blood: ⬤ Many (second most common WBC component of blood)
- Bone Marrow: ⚙ Scattered
- Lymph Node: B-cells mainly in follicular areas and T-cells mainly in Interfollicular areas

↔ May Resemble
- Blast {p. 140}
- Orthochromic Normoblast {p. 12}
- Plasma Cell (mature) {p. 67}
- Reactive Lymphocyte {p. 137}
- Monocyte {p. 144}

ᴰˣ Differential Diagnoses
- Increased number of normal (non-neoplastic) lymphocytes may be associated with:
  - Infection (viral, fungal, and some bacterial)
  - Autoimmune disorders

⚙ Classic Immunophenotype
T-cells:
  - CD2 ➕, CD3 ➕, CD5 ➕, CD7 ➕
  - Subset CD4 ➕
  - Subset CD8 ➕
B-cells:
  - CD19 ➕, CD20 ➕
  - Subset kappa ➕
  - Subset lambda ➕

Miscellaneous: Normal lymphocytes are the second most common WBCs in the blood (after neutrophils).

🜛 Lymphocyte-Abnormal

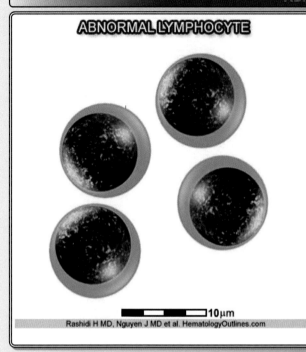

ABNORMAL LYMPHOCYTE

10μm

Rashidi H MD, Nguyen J MD et al. HematologyOutlines.com

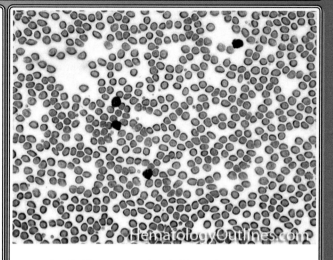

The WBCs seen in this field are lymphocytes.

🔬 Microscopic Features
- *Range in size from slightly (1.5X) larger than a mature RBC to 2-4X larger than a RBC*
- High nuclear-to-cytoplasmic ratio but with a round mature nucleus (clumped chromatin)
- Nucleoli are absent in most
- Cytoplasm is scant, light blue and lacks granules

⚠ Frequency in Tissues
- Peripheral Blood: ⊘ None
- Bone Marrow: ⊘ None
- Lymph Node: ⊘ None

↔ May Resemble
- Blast {p. 140}
- Orthochromic Normoblast {p. 12}
- Plasma Cell (mature) {p. 67}
- Reactive Lymphocyte {p. 137}
- Monocyte {p. 144}

ᴅx Differential Diagnoses
- If increased in blood, lymph node or bone marrow:
  - Infection
  - Neoplastic (mature B or T-cell lymphoma or leukemia)

⚙ Classic Immunophenotype
- Can be T-, B-, or NK-cells (usually with some immunophenotypic aberrancy)

Miscellaneous: It is not possible to distinguish T-cells and B-cells based on morphology alone.

ABNORMAL

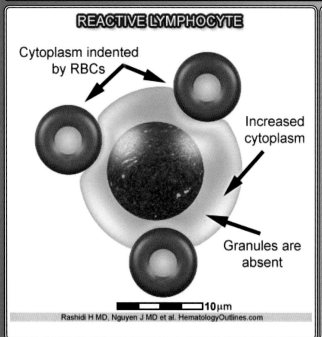

REACTIVE LYMPHOCYTE

Cytoplasm indented by RBCs

Increased cytoplasm

Granules are absent

10μm

Rashidi H MD, Nguyen J MD et al. HematologyOutlines.com

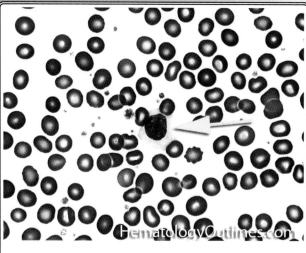

Notice the cytoplasm is wrapping around surrounding RBCs.

🔬 Microscopic Features
- 2-4X larger than a mature RBC
- Increased amount of light blue cytoplasm
- Nucleoli usually absent
- *Cytoplasm is usually indented by surrounding red blood cells*
- Granules are usually absent (as opposed to LGL)

⚠ Frequency in Tissues
- Peripheral Blood: ○ Rare to none
- Bone Marrow: ⊘ None
- Lymph Node: ⊘ None

↔ May Resemble
- Lymphocyte (mature) {p. 135}
- Myeloblast {p. 123}
- Monocyte {p. 144}
- Large Granular Lymphocyte {p. 138}

Dx Differential Diagnoses
- ↑ Increased numbers in blood may be due to:
  - ○ Epstein-Barr virus infection (infectious mononucleosis)
  - ○ CMV infection
  - ○ Other viral Infections
  - ○ Drug reaction
  - ○ Chronic inflammatory disorders (e.g.systemic lupus erythematosis, rheumatoid arthritis)

⚙ Classic Immunophenotype
Usually are CD8 ➕ T-cells:
- CD2 ➕ and CD3 ➕
- CD8 ➕
- CD4 ➖
- CD5 ➕
- CD7 ➕

Miscellaneous: Increased numbers may be seen in some viral infections (e.g. EBV mononucleosis).

🩸 Large Granular Lymphocyte (LGL)

LARGE GRANULAR LYMPHOCYTE

Abundant light blue cytoplasm

Absent nucleoli

Round, mature nucleus

Pink/red granules

10μm

Rashidi H MD, Nguyen J MD et al. HematologyOutlines.com

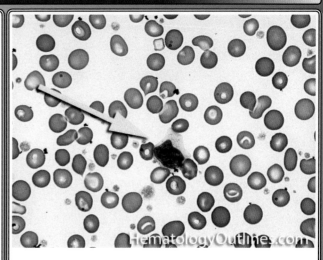

The yellow arrow points to the large granular lymphocyte. Note the large reddish granules in the cytoplasm.

🔬 Microscopic Features
- 2-4X larger than a mature RBC
- Low nuclear-to-cytoplasmic ratio because of the increased cytoplasm
- Round-to-convoluted nuclear border with mature chromatin (clumped chromatin)
- Nucleoli are absent
- Cytoplasm is abundant and light blue
- ***Pink/red granules seen within the cytoplasm (hence the term "granular")***

⚠ Frequency in Tissues
- Peripheral Blood: ○ Rare to ⊘ None
- Bone Marrow: ⊘ None
- Lymph Node: ⊘ None

↔ May Resemble
- Reactive Lymphocyte {p. 137}
- Monocyte {p. 144}
- Promyelocyte {p. 124}

℞x Differential Diagnoses
- Infection/inflammatory
- Neoplastic (LGL leukemia)

⚙ Classic Immunophenotype
- CD2 ⊞
- CD3 ⊞
- CD4 ⊝
- CD8 ⊞
- CD5 ⊞
- CD7 ⊞
- CD16 ⊞
- CD56 ⊞ / ⊝
- CD57 ⊞

Miscellaneous: One must rule out reactive conditions (e.g. infection, etc.) before considering LGL leukemia as a diagnosis.

🩸 Chronic Lymphocytic Leukemia (CLL)

ABNORMAL LYMPHOCYTE

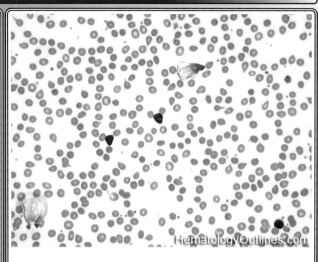

10µm

Rashidi H MD, Nguyen J MD et al. HematologyOutlines.com

Notice the WBCs are mostly small lymphocytes with scattered smudge cells.

🔬 Microscopic Features
- Increased number of small to intermediate sized lymphocytes in the peripheral blood (usually >5000/microL absolute count)
- Minimal nuclear membrane irregularities
- Nucleoli are absent
- *Background smudge cells (smeared, partially broken up cells) are common but not specific to CLL*

⚠ Frequency in Tissues
- Peripheral Blood: ⊘ None
- Bone Marrow: ⊘ None
- Lymph Node: ⊘ None

↔ May Resemble
- Lymphocyte (mature) {p. 135}
- Reactive Lymphocyte {p. 137}
- Mantle Cell Leukemia {p. 81} (mantle cell lymphoma in blood)

℞x Differential Diagnoses
- Reactive lymphocytosis
- Mantle cell leukemia
- Other mature B or T-cell leukemias
- Monoclonal B-cell lymphocytosis

⚙ Classic Immunophenotype
- CD19 ➕
- CD20 **dim** ➕
- FMC7 ➖
- CD5 ➕
- CD23 ➕
- BCL1 ➖
- Dim surface light chain (kappa or lambda) restricted

Miscellaneous: CLL is a low grade non-Hodgkin B-cell leukemia mostly seen in the elderly population. In tissue it is called small lymphocytic lymphoma (SLL).

🩸 Lymphoblasts in ALL

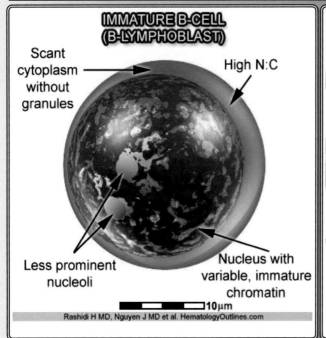

IMMATURE B-CELL
(B-LYMPHOBLAST)

Scant cytoplasm without granules

High N:C

Less prominent nucleoli

Nucleus with variable, immature chromatin

10μm

Rashidi H MD, Nguyen J MD et al. HematologyOutlines.com

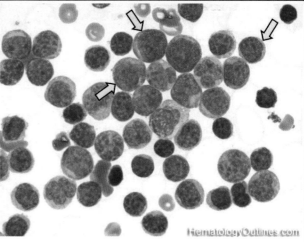

Notice the open chromatin and prominent nucleoli in the large cells.

🔬 Microscopic Features
- 3-4X larger than a mature RBC
- *High nuclear-to-cytoplasmic ratio*
- Round nucleus with immature chromatin (not clumped)
- Prominent nucleoli
- Cytoplasm is scant, light blue and lacks granules

⚠ Frequency in Tissues
- Peripheral Blood: ⊘ None
- Bone Marrow: ⊘ None
- Lymph Node: ⊘ None

↔ May Resemble
- Myeloblast {p. 123}
- Pronormoblast {p. 9}
- Monoblast {p. 38}
- Immature B-cell (hematogone) {p. 62}
- Reactive Lymphocyte {p. 137}

Dx Differential Diagnoses
- If in blood or increased in marrow or tissue:
  - B-Lymphoblastic leukemia (B-ALL)
  - T-Lymphoblastic leukemia (T-ALL)
  - CML lymphoblastic blast crisis

⚙ Classic Immunophenotype
- B-lymphoblasts
  - CD19 ⊞ and CD10 ⊞
  - CD20 ⊟
  - CD34 ⊞ and TdT ⊞
  - Kappa ⊟ and lambda ⊟
- T-lymphoblasts
  - CD2 ⊞/⊟, CD3 ⊞, CD5 ⊞/⊟ CD7 ⊞/⊟
  - CD4 ⊞/⊟, CD8 ⊞/⊟
  - CD34 ⊞ and TdT ⊞

Miscellaneous: Blasts cells cannot be reliably distinguished from each other based on morphology alone. The exception are blasts with Auer rod(s) which are unique to abnormal myeloblasts and abnormal promyelocytes as noted in some AMLs and APL.

📓 **Note**: Abnormal lymphoblasts can show immunophenotypic abberancies (e.g. gain of myeloid markers).

🩸 Hairy Cell Leukemia

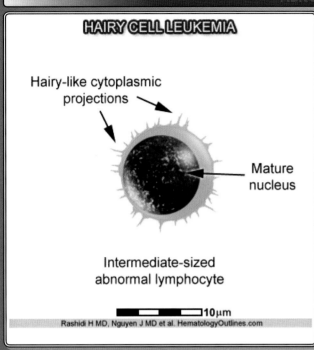

HAIRY CELL LEUKEMIA

Hairy-like cytoplasmic projections

Mature nucleus

Intermediate-sized abnormal lymphocyte

├─────────10μm

Rashidi H MD, Nguyen J MD et al. HematologyOutlines.com

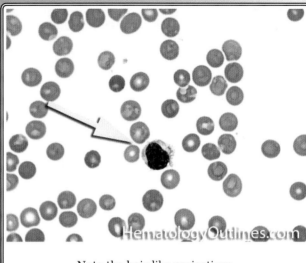

Note the hair-like projections.

🔬 Microscopic Features
- *Peripheral blood smear shows lymphocytes with hair-like cytoplasmic projections*
- Abnormal lymphocytes with hair-like projections are intermediate in size
- Lacks a nucleolus
- The neoplastic cells typically involve the red pulp areas of the spleen (as opposed to splenic marginal zone lymphoma which involves the white pulp)

⚠ Frequency in Tissues
- Peripheral Blood: ⊘ None
- Bone Marrow: ⊘ None
- Lymph Node: ⊘ None

↔ May Resemble
- Splenic Marginal Zone Lymphoma {p. 88}
- Reactive Lymphocyte {p. 137}
- Chronic Lymphocytic Leukemia (CLL) {p. 139}

ᴅx Differential Diagnoses
- Splenic marginal zone lymphoma
- Reactive lymphocytosis
- Chronic lymphocytic leukemia (CLL)

⚙ Classic Immunophenotype
- CD19 ⊞ and CD20 ⊞
- CD5 ⊖
- CD10 ⊖
- CD103 ⊞
- CD11c ⊞
- CD25 ⊞
- Annexin A1 ⊞

Miscellaneous: Many cases present with splenomegaly, cytopenia or pancytopenia (many with monocytopenia), and a dry bone marrow aspirate (dry tap). Most also carry the BRAF V600E mutation.

🩸 Sézary Cell

SÉZARY CELL

Scant light blue cytoplasm

Nucleoli usually absent

Irregular nuclear membrane
(cerebriform nucleus: looks like "brain")

■□□□10µm

Rashidi H MD, Nguyen J MD et al. HematologyOutlines.com

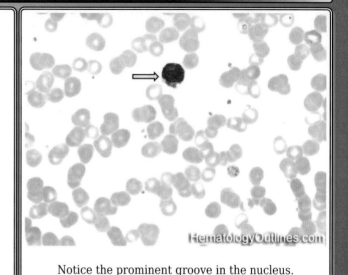

Notice the prominent groove in the nucleus.

🔬 Microscopic Features
- Small to intermediate sized lymphocytes
- *Irregular nuclear membrane (cerebriform nucleus: looks like a "brain")*
- Nucleoli are usually absent
- Scant amount of light blue cytoplasm

⚠ Frequency in Tissues
- Peripheral Blood: ⊘ None
- Bone Marrow: ⊘ None
- Lymph Node: ⊘ None

↔ May Resemble
- Lymphocyte (mature) {p. 135}
- Polychromatophilic RBC {p. 92}

℞x Differential Diagnoses
- Sézary syndrome
- Other T-cell lymphoproliferative disorders with blood involvement
- Infection/inflammation

⚙ Classic Immunophenotype
- CD2 ➕/ ➖
- CD3 ➕
- CD4 ➕
- CD5 ➕/ ➖
- CD8 ➖
- CD7 ➖
- CD26 ➖

Miscellaneous: Sézary syndrome refers to a triad of erythroderma (likely with skin involvement by the underlying T-cell lymphoma), lymphadenopathy, and circulating abnormal neoplastic T-cell in the blood.

Monocyte Maturation Overview Diagram

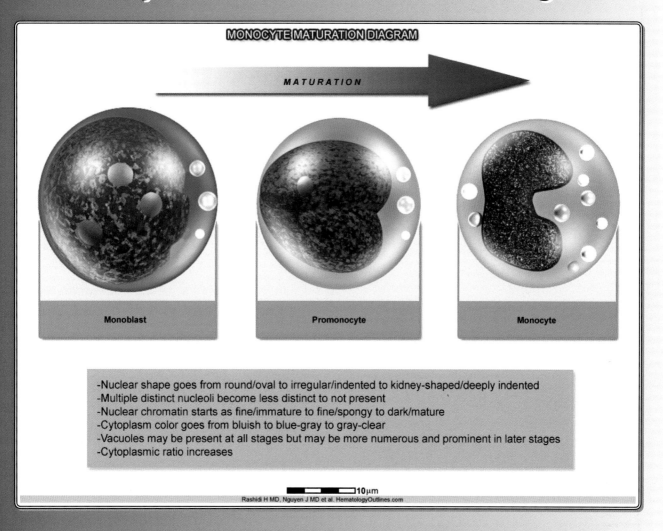

MONOCYTE MATURATION DIAGRAM

MATURATION

| Monoblast | Promonocyte | Monocyte |

-Nuclear shape goes from round/oval to irregular/indented to kidney-shaped/deeply indented
-Multiple distinct nucleoli become less distinct to not present
-Nuclear chromatin starts as fine/immature to fine/spongy to dark/mature
-Cytoplasm color goes from bluish to blue-gray to gray-clear
-Vacuoles may be present at all stages but may be more numerous and prominent in later stages
-Cytoplasmic ratio increases

10μm

Rashidi H MD, Nguyen J MD et al. HematologyOutlines.com

Stages of maturation go from monoblast to promonocyte to monocyte to macrophage. The nucleus is oval, horseshoe or kidney shaped and is usually eccentric. The chromatin is less dense than in lymphocytes. Monoblasts and promonocytes are rare and predominantly contained to the bone marrow while mature monocytes are mostly seen in peripheral blood. As mature monocytes leave the peripheral blood and enter tissue, they become macrophages/histiocytes. Monoblasts and promonocytes contain nucleoli (a sign of immaturity), while the mature monocytes and macrophages lack nucleoli (since they are mature).

◊ Monocyte

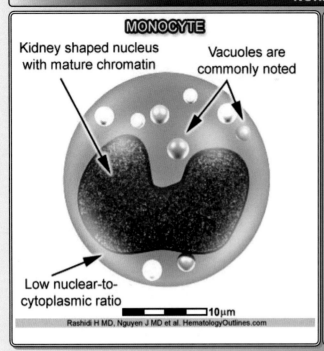

MONOCYTE

Kidney shaped nucleus with mature chromatin

Vacuoles are commonly noted

Low nuclear-to-cytoplasmic ratio

10μm

Rashidi H MD, Nguyen J MD et al. HematologyOutlines.com

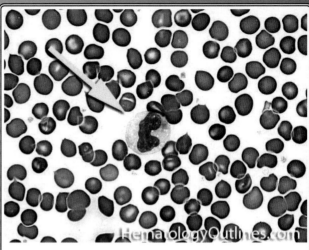

The yellow arrow points to the mature monocyte. Notice the kidney shaped nucleus and cytoplasmic vacuoles.

🔬 Microscopic Features
- 3-4X larger than a mature RBC
- Lower nuclear-to-cytoplasmic ratio because of increased cytoplasm
- *Kidney shaped indented nucleus with mature chromatin (clumped)*
- Nucleoli are absent
- Cytoplasm is abundant, gray to pale blue and with rare to no granules
- Vacuoles are commonly noted in cytoplasm

⚠ Frequency in Tissues
- Peripheral Blood: 3rd most common WBC (after neutrophils and lymphocytes)
- Bone Marrow: ✪ Scattered (some in the form of histiocytes/macrophages)
- Lymph Node: ✪ Scattered (some in the form of histiocytes/macrophages)

↔ May Resemble
- Reactive Lymphocyte {p. 137}
- Myelocyte {p. 125}
- Metamyelocyte {p. 126}
- Band Neutrophil {p. 127}
- Promonocyte {p. 39}
- Monoblast {p. 145}

Dx Differential Diagnoses
- Chronic myelomonocytic leukemia
- Autoimmune disorders (sometimes)
- Chronic infections (e.g. CMV, tuberculosis, etc.)

✿ Classic Immunophenotype
- CD45 ➕ with intermediate SSC (side light scatter)
- CD14 ➕
- CD4 **dim** ➕
- CD64 ➕

Miscellaneous: Monocytes leave the blood and enter tissue to become macrophages/histiocytes.

🩸 Monoblast

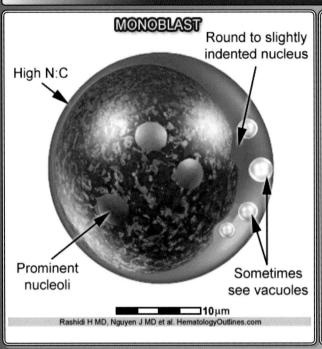

MONOBLAST

High N:C

Round to slightly indented nucleus

Prominent nucleoli

Sometimes see vacuoles

10μm

Rashidi H MD, Nguyen J MD et al. HematologyOutlines.com

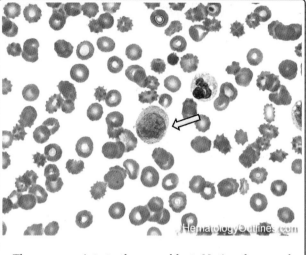

The arrow points to the monoblast. Notice the round nucleus and the prominent nucleolus.

🔬 Microscopic Features
- 3-4X larger than a mature RBC
- *High nuclear-to-cytoplasmic ratio*
- Round to slightly indented nucleus with immature chromatin (not clumped)
- Prominent nucleoli
- Cytoplasm is scant, gray to pale blue (more cytoplasm than a myeloblast) and with rare or absent granules
- Vacuoles are rare but sometimes noted in cytoplasm

⚠️ Frequency in Tissues
- Peripheral Blood: ⊘ None
- Bone Marrow: 1%
- Lymph Node: ⊘ None

↔ May Resemble
- Promonocyte {p. 39}
- Myeloblast {p. 123}
- Lymphoblast {p. 65}
- Pronormoblast {p. 9}
- Mature Monocyte {p. 144}
- Reactive Lymphocyte {p. 137}
- Lymphoma cell (e.g. Leukemic phase of Burkitt lymphoma)
- Carcinoma cell

Dx Differential Diagnoses
- ↑ Increased in:
  - Acute monocytic leukemia
  - Acute myelomonocytic leukemia (AMML)
  - Chronic myelomonocytic leukemia (CMML)

⚙️ Classic Immunophenotype
- CD34 ➕/➖, CD117 ➕/➖
- HLA-DR ➕
- CD13 ➕ and CD33 ➕
- CD64 ➕
- CD4 **dim** ➕
- CD14 ➖

Miscellaneous: In monocyte-differentiated leukemias, the total blast count is equal to monoblasts + promonocytes (since promonocytes are considered in this instance to be equivalent to blasts).

🔹 Promonocyte

ABNORMAL

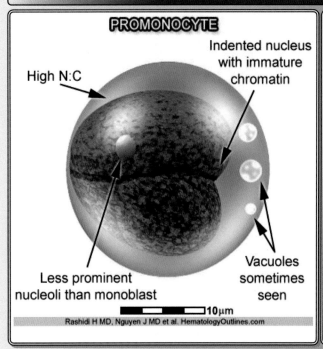

PROMONOCYTE

High N:C

Indented nucleus with immature chromatin

Less prominent nucleoli than monoblast

Vacuoles sometimes seen

10μm

Rashidi H MD, Nguyen J MD et al. HematologyOutlines.com

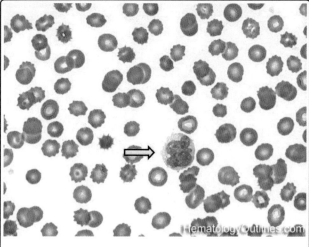

The yellow arrow points to the promonocyte. Note the prominent nucleolus.

🔬 Microscopic Features
- 3-4X larger than a mature RBC
- **Round indented nucleus with immature chromatin (not clumped; slightly more mature than a monoblast)**
- Prominent nucleoli (less prominent than monoblast)
- Cytoplasm is scant but more than myeloblasts, and is gray to pale blue with rare or no granules
- Vacuoles maybe sometimes noted in the cytoplasm

⚠ Frequency in Tissues
- Peripheral Blood: ⊘ None
- Bone Marrow: 1%
- Lymph Node: ⊘ None

↔ May Resemble
- Monoblast {p. 145}
- Myeloblast {p. 123}
- Mature Monocyte {p. 144}
- Reactive Lymphocyte {p. 137}
- Lymphoma cell (e.g. Leukemic phase of Burkitt lymphoma)
- Carcinoma cell

Dx Differential Diagnoses
- Acute monocytic Leukemia
- Acute myelomonocytic leukemia (AMML)
- Chronic myelomonocytic leukemia (CMML)
- Infection/inflammation

⚙ Classic Immunophenotype
- CD34 ⊖, CD117 ⊖ / ⊕, HLA-DR ⊕
- CD13 ⊕, CD15 ⊕, CD33 ⊕
- CD64 ⊕
- CD14 ⊖/⊕
- CD4 **dim** ⊕

Miscellaneous: Promonocytes count as blasts when looking for total blast count. In myeloid leukemias with monocytic differentiation, the total blast count is equal to monoblasts + promonocytes.

⬤ Increased Mature Monocytes

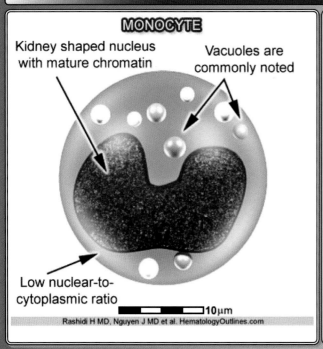

MONOCYTE

Kidney shaped nucleus with mature chromatin

Vacuoles are commonly noted

Low nuclear-to-cytoplasmic ratio

10µm

Rashidi H MD, Nguyen J MD et al. HematologyOutlines.com

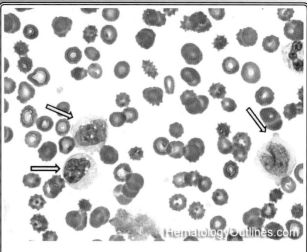

The yellow arrows point out the increase in monocytes in the field of view. Notice the lack of a nucleolus in these mature monocytes.

🔬 Microscopic Features
- 3-4X larger than a mature RBC
- Lower nuclear-to-cytoplasmic ratio because of increased cytoplasm
- *Kidney-shaped indented nucleus with mature chromatin (clumped)*
- Nucleoli is absent
- Cytoplasm is abundant, gray to pale blue and lacks granules
- Vacuoles are commonly noted in cytoplasm

⚠ Frequency in Tissues
- Peripheral Blood: 3rd most common WBC (after neutrophils and lymphocytes)
- Bone Marrow: ⚽ Scattered (some as histiocytes/macrophages)
- Lymph Node: ⚽ Scattered (some as histiocytes/macrophages)

↔ May Resemble
- Reactive Lymphocyte {p. 137}
- Myelocyte {p. 125}
- Metamyelocyte {p. 126}
- Band Neutrophil {p. 127}
- Promonocyte {p. 146}
- Monoblast {p. 145}

ᴅx Differential Diagnoses
- Chronic myelomonocytic leukemia
- Chronic neutropenia
- Autoimmune (sometimes)
- Chronic infections (e.g. CMV, tuberculosis, etc.)

⚙ Classic Immunophenotype
- CD45 ➕
- CD34 ➖, CD1147 ➖, and HLA-DR ➕
- Intermediate SSC (side light scatter)
- CD14 ➕ and CD64 ➕
- CD13 ➕, CD15 ➕, and CD33 ➕
- CD4 **dim** ➕

Miscellaneous: Increased monocytes can be associated with many processes including, but not limited to, infectious etiologies.

⬤ Eosinophil (Mature)

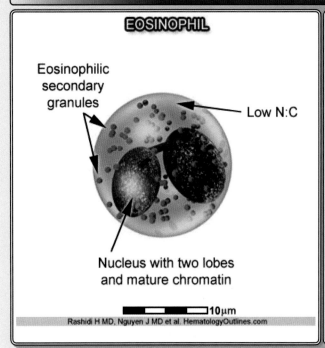

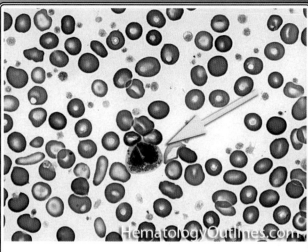

The arrow points to the mature eosinophil. Note the bilobed nucleus and prominent red granules.

🔬 Microscopic Features

- 2-3X larger than a mature RBC
- Low nuclear-to-cytoplasmic ratio (more cytoplasm than nucleus)
- *Nucleus is mature and usually with 2 lobes connected by thin chromatin filament*
- Nucleoli are absent
- More cytoplasm with only secondary granules
- *Secondary (specific) granules are eosinophilic (red-orange color)*

⚠ Frequency in Tissues

- Peripheral Blood: ✲ Scattered (4th most common WBC in blood, after neutrophils, lymphocytes and monocytes)
- Bone Marrow: ◯ Rare
- Lymph Node: ◯ Rare to ⊘ None

↔ May Resemble

- Segmented Neutrophil {p. 128}
- Pseudo-Pelger Huet Neutrophil {p. 132}
- Band Neutrophil {p. 127}
- Neutrophil With Toxic Granules {p. 131}
- Promyelocyte {p. 124}
- Basophil {p. 151}

℞x Differential Diagnoses

- Allergy-related (e.g. Asthma)
- Drug reactions
- Invasive parasitic infections
- Myeloproliferative neoplasms
- Hodgkin's and non-Hodgkin's lymphomas
- Autoimmune disorders (some)

⚙ Classic Immunophenotype

- CD45 **dim** ✚
- CD10 ⊖, CD14 ⊖, CD64 ⊖, HLA-DR ⊖
- High SSC (side light scatter)
- CD13 **dim** ✚, CD33 ✚, CD11b ✚, CD11c ✚
- CD16 ⊖
- CD15 **dim** ✚

Miscellaneous: Increased amounts are commonly associated with: drugs, allergy, infection (especially invasive multicellular parasites), neoplasms (e.g. myeloid neoplasms such as some AMLs or MPNs), and idiopathic causes.

💧 Eosinophil (Increased)

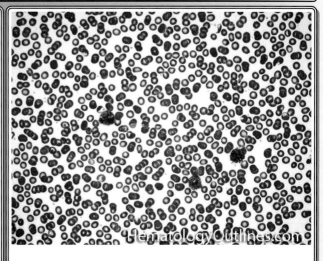

EOSINOPHIL

Eosinophilic secondary granules

Low N:C

Nucleus with two lobes and mature chromatin

10μm

Rashidi H MD, Nguyen J MD et al. HematologyOutlines.com

Three eosinophils are seen among many red blood cells in this field of view.

🔬 Microscopic Features
- 2-3X larger than a mature RBC
- Low nuclear-to-cytoplasmic ratio (more cytoplasm than nucleus)
- *Nucleus is mature and usually with 2 lobes connected by thin chromatin filament*
- Nucleoli are absent
- More cytoplasm with only secondary granules
- *Secondary (specific) granules are eosinophilic (red-orange color)*

⚠ Frequency in Tissues
- Peripheral Blood: ✹ Scattered (4th most common WBC in blood, after neutrophils, lymphocytes and monocytes)
- Bone Marrow: ○ Rare
- Lymph Node: ○ Rare to ⊘ None

↔ May Resemble
- Segmented Neutrophil {p. 128}
- Pseudo-Pelger Huet Neutrophil {p. 132}
- Band Neutrophil {p. 127}
- Neutrophil With Toxic Granules {p. 131}
- Promyelocyte {p. 124}
- Basophil {p. 151}

Dx Differential Diagnoses
- Allergy-related (e.g. Asthma)
- Drug reactions
- Invasive parasitic infections
- Myeloproliferative neoplasms
- Hodgkin's and non-Hodgkin's lymphomas
- Autoimmune disorders (some)

⚙ Classic Immunophenotype
- CD45 **dim** ⊞
- HLA-DR ⊖, CD10 ⊖
- CD14 ⊖, CD64 ⊖
- High SSC (side light scatter)
- CD13 **dim** ⊞, CD15 **dim** ⊞, CD33 ⊞
- CD11b ⊞, CD11c ⊞
- CD16 ⊖

Miscellaneous: Increased amounts are commonly associated with: drugs, allergy, infection (especially invasive multicellular parasites), neoplasms (e.g. myeloid neoplasms such as some AMLs or MPNs), and idiopathic causes.

Dysplastic Eosinophil

DYSPLASTIC EOSINOPHIL

Low N:C

Abnormal
secondary
granules

Mature nucleus;
some may have 1 lobe
or more than 2 lobes

10µm

Rashidi H MD, Nguyen J MD et al. HematologyOutlines.com

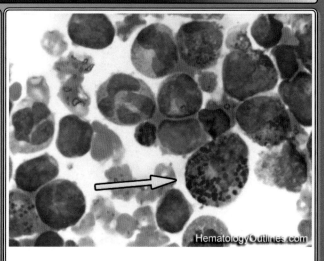

The yellow arrow points to an abnormal eosinophil with abnormal basophilic-like granules.

Microscopic Features
- 2-3X larger than a mature RBC
- Low nuclear-to-cytoplasmic ratio (more cytoplasm than nucleus)
- Nucleus is mature and usually with 2 lobes connected by thin chromatin (some have 1 lobe or >2 lobes)
- Nucleoli are absent
- *More cytoplasm with abnormal secondary granules (usually darker like basophilic granules)*
- The granules are heterogenous and vacuoules may occasionally be noted as well

Frequency in Tissues
- Peripheral Blood: ⊘ None
- Bone Marrow: ⊘ None
- Lymph Node: ⊘ None

May Resemble
- Eosinophil {p. 148}
- Basophil {p. 151}
- Neutrophil (mature) {p. 128}
- Pseudo-Pelger Huet Neutrophil {p. 132}
- Band Neutrophil {p. 127}

Differential Diagnoses
- Certain AMLs such as AML with inv 16 or t(16;16)
- Certain myeloproliferative neoplasms
- Certain myelodysplastic syndromes (MDS)

Classic Immunophenotype
- CD45 **dim** ⊞ with high SSC (side light scatter)
- CD13 **dim** ⊞
- CD16 ⊖
- CD15 **dim** ⊞
- May have some immunophenotypic variability compared to normal eosinophils

Miscellaneous: AML with inv16 or t(16;16) was also known as AML-M4Eo (which stood for an AML with monocytic differentiation and abnormal eosinophils). The gene involved is CBF-B.

💧 Basophil (Mature)

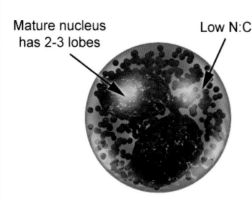

BASOPHIL

Mature nucleus has 2-3 lobes

Low N:C

Nucleus may be obscured by numerous basophilic secondary granules

⊢━━━━⊣10µm

Rashidi H MD, Nguyen J MD et al. HematologyOutlines.com

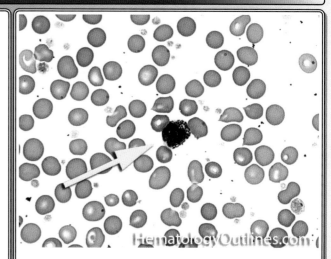

The arrow points to the basophil. Notice the granules obscuring the nucleus.

🔬 Microscopic Features
- 2-3X larger than a mature RBC
- Low nuclear-to-cytoplasmic ratio (more cytoplasm than nucleus)
- Nucleus is mature and usually with 2-3 lobes connected by a thin chromatin filament
- Nucleoli are absent and more cytoplasm with only secondary granules
- *Secondary (specific) granules are basophilic (blue-violet color) and obscure the underlying nucleus*

⚠ Frequency in Tissues
- Peripheral Blood: ○ Rare (5th most common WBC)
- Bone Marrow: ○ Rare
- Lymph Node: ⊘ None

↔ May Resemble
- Eosinophil {p. 148}
- Segmented Neutrophil {p. 128}
- Pseudo-Pelger Huet Neutrophil {p. 132}
- Neutrophil With Toxic Granules {p. 131}
- Promyelocyte {p. 124}
- Mast cell (see in Glossary)

℞x Differential Diagnoses
- CML accelerated phase AML (rare variants)
- Infection (e.g. varicella)
- Hypersensitivity reactions

⚙ Classic Immunophenotype
- CD34 ⊖ and CD117 ⊖
- CD45 **dim** ⊕ (less bright than lymphocytes)
- Low SSC (side light scatter)
- CD11b ⊕ and CD13 ⊕
- CD22 ⊕, CD25 **dim** ⊕, CD33 ⊕
- CD38 ⊕⊕ and CD123 ⊕⊕
- CD16 ⊖ and CD15 ⊖

Miscellaneous: Increased basophils may be associated with some myeloid neoplasms such as CML, some infections or some hypersensitivity reactions. Basophils and mast cells are distinct from one another but share some similar morphologic and functional aspects. As opposed to basophils which can be seen in the peripheral blood, mast cells are only seen in tissue and absent from the peripheral blood. Additionally, the nucleus of the mast cell is usually round and not segmented as opposed to the basophil's segmented (usually bi-lobed) nucleus. The granules of basophils are more heterogenous and overlap the nucleus while the granules of mast cells are more uniform and less often cover the nucleus.

🜄 Basophils (Increased)

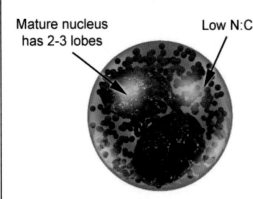

BASOPHIL

Mature nucleus has 2-3 lobes

Low N:C

Nucleus may be obscured by numerous basophilic secondary granules

10μm

Rashidi H MD, Nguyen J MD et al. HematologyOutlines.com

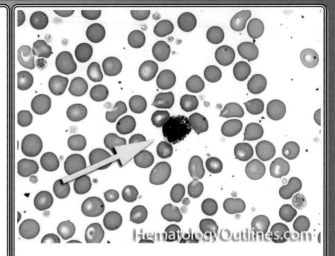

The yellow arrow points to a basophil. Basophils are rarely seen in a normal blood smear.

🔬 Microscopic Features
- 2-3X larger than a mature RBC
- Low nuclear-to-cytoplasmic ratio (more cytoplasm than nucleus)
- Nucleus is mature and usually with 2-3 lobes connected by a thin chromatin filament
- Nucleoli are absent
- More cytoplasm with only secondary granules
- *Secondary (specific) granules are basophilic (blue-violet color) and obscure the underlying nucleus*

⚠ Frequency in Tissues
- Peripheral Blood: Very Rare (5th most common WBC in blood, after neutrophils, lymphocytes, monocytes, and Eosinophils)
- Bone Marrow: ○ Rare
- Lymph Node: ⊘ None

↔ May Resemble
- Eosinophil {p. 148}
- Segmented Neutrophil {p. 128}
- Pseudo-Pelger Huet Neutrophil {p. 132}
- Band Neutrophil {p. 127}
- Neutrophil With Toxic Granules {p. 131}
- Promyelocyte {p. 124}
- Mast cell (see in Glossary)

Dx Differential Diagnoses
- Chronic myeloid leukemia (CML) accelerated phase
- Acute myeloid leukemia (AML, rare variants)
- Infection (e.g. varicella)
- Hypersensitivity reactions (sometimes)

⚙ Classic Immunophenotype
- CD34 ⊖ and CD117 ⊖
- CD45 **dim** ⊕ (less bright than lymphocytes)
- Low SSC (side light scatter)
- CD11b ⊕ and CD13 ⊕
- CD22 ⊕, CD25 **dim** ⊕, CD33 ⊕
- CD38 ⊕⊕ and CD123 ⊕⊕
- CD16 ⊖ and CD15 ⊖

Miscellaneous: Increased basophils may be associated with some myeloid neoplasms such as CML, or some infections or some hypersensitivity reactions.

⬤ Platelets

PLATELETS

Wide variation in shape and size, usually round or elliptical

Clear or slightly blue-gray cytoplasm

On high power, can see purple or red granules (dispersed or centrally aggregated)

━━━━━10μm

Rashidi H MD, Nguyen J MD et al. HematologyOutlines.com

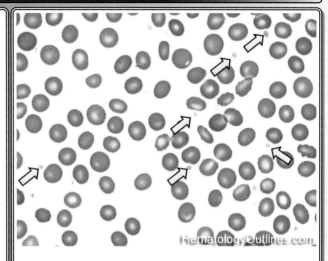

The yellow arrows point to the platelets.

🔬 Microscopic Features
- *Most are 1/5 to 1/3 the size of a normal red blood cell*
- They are typically round with a blue-gray cytoplasm
- Cytoplasm has purple/blue granules

⚠ Frequency in Tissues
- Peripheral Blood: ⬤ Many
- Bone Marrow: ✪ Scattered
- Lymph Node: ⊘ None

↔ May Resemble
- Schistocyte {p. 100}
- Stain precipitate
- Malaria Infection {p. 115}
- Babesia Infection {p. 116}

Dx Differential Diagnoses
↑ Increased in:
- Iron deficiency anemia
- Acute or chronic inflammation
- Myeloproliferative neoplasms
- Drug reaction / exercise

↓ Decreased in:
- Microangiopathic hemolytic anemias
- Malignancy with marrow infiltration
- Drug induced infection (e.g. sepsis leading to DIC)
- Autoimmune (e.g. ITP)
- Nutritional deficiencies
- Splenic sequestration
- Hereditary causes

⚙ Classic Immunophenotype
- CD41 ➕
- CD42 ➕
- CD61 ➕

Miscellaneous: Platelets are the smallest cellular fragments noted on a peripheral blood smear.

◈ Platelet Satellitosis

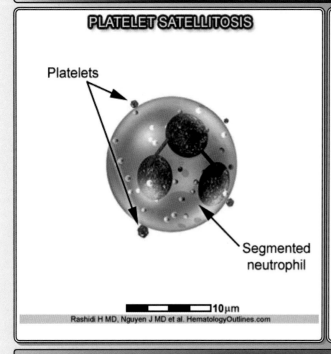

PLATELET SATELLITOSIS

Platelets

Segmented neutrophil

10µm

Rashidi H MD, Nguyen J MD et al. HematologyOutlines.com

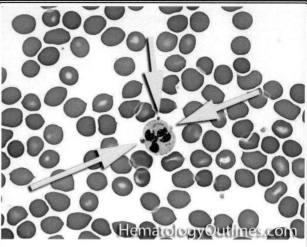

The granulocyte is surrounded by a few platelets.

🔬 Microscopic Features
- *Small platelets or platelet aggregates surrounding the cell membrane of a neutrophil or monocyte*

⚠ Frequency in Tissues
- Peripheral Blood: ○ Rare to ⊘ None
- Bone Marrow: ○ Rare to ⊘ None
- Lymph Node: ⊘ None

↔ May Resemble
- Stain artifact
- Monocyte {p. 144}
- Neutrophil {p. 128}

℞x Differential Diagnoses
- EDTA-induced
- Autoimmune-disorders
- Pregnancy

⚙ Classic Immunophenotype
- CD41 ➕
- CD42 ➕
- CD61 ➕

Miscellaneous: As a result of the platelets attaching to the surface of neutrophils or monocytes, the platelet count measured by an automated instrument for a complete blood count (CBC) could become falsely decreased (pseudo-thrombocytopenia).

🩸 Giant Platelets

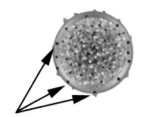

GIANT PLATELET

Larger than normal RBC

Purple or red granules

⊐10μm

Rashidi H MD, Nguyen J MD et al. HematologyOutlines.com

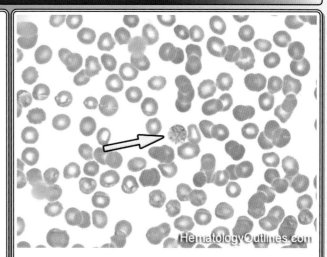

The platelet at the yellow arrow is larger than the mature normal RBC.

🔬 Microscopic Features
- *Larger than normal red blood cells*
- Usually looks like a very large platelet and has platelet granules in the cytoplasm
- It may be confused sometimes for a lymphocyte

⚠ Frequency in Tissues
- Peripheral Blood: ⊘ None
- Bone Marrow: ⊘ None
- Lymph Node: ⊘ None

↔ May Resemble
- Lymphocyte (mature) {p. 135}
- Polychromatophilic RBC {p. 92}
- Malaria Infection {p. 115}
- Babesia Infection {p. 116}

Dx Differential Diagnoses
- ↑ Increased numbers may be see in:
  - Myeloid neoplasms (e.g. MDS, acute leukemia or myeloproliferative neoplasms)
  - Post-splenectomy patients
  - Leukemoid reaction
  - Some rare inherited conditions (e.g.May-Hegglin anomaly, Bernard-Soulier syndrome, etc.)

⚙ Classic Immunophenotype
- CD41 ⊞
- CD42 ⊞
- CD61 ⊞

Miscellaneous: The term giant platelet is used if the size is greater than that of a normal red blood cell, and the term large platelet can be used to describe those bigger than normal platelets and less than the size of a normal red blood cell.

⬥ Agranular Platelets

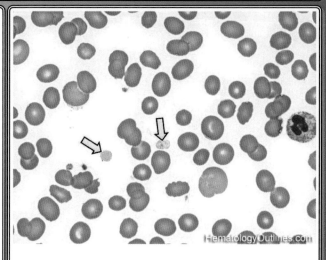

AGRANULAR PLATELETS

10μm

Rashidi H MD, Nguyen J MD et al. HematologyOutlines.com

Notice the pale (due to lack or decreased granules) appearance of the platelets.

🔬 Microscopic Features
- Smaller than a normal red blood cell (usually much smaller, similar to normal platelets)
- *Lacks the darker staining platelet granules*

⚠ Frequency in Tissues
- Peripheral Blood: ◯ Rare to ⊘ None
- Bone Marrow: ◯ Rare to ⊘ None
- Lymph Node: ⊘ None

↔ May Resemble
- Stain precipitate
- Malaria Infection {p. 115}
- Babesia Infection {p. 116}

Dx Differential Diagnoses
- ↑ Increased numbers may be seen in:
  - Myeloid neoplasms (e.g. MDS, acute leukemia or myeloproliferative neoplasms)
  - Gray platelet syndrome (alpha storage pool disease)

⚙ Classic Immunophenotype
- CD41 ⊞
- CD42 ⊞/⊖
- CD61 ⊞

Miscellaneous: Lack of platelet granules may be indicative of an underlying abnormality of the platelets such as, but not limited to, the inability of producing certain platelet granules.

Hematology Glossary

Abciximab	A monoclonal antibody (immunoglobulin) that binds glycoprotein IIb/IIIa on platelets and inhibits platelet function/aggregation. This particular drug has been used in percutaneous transluminal coronary artery stenting procedures. Note: Drugs ending with "mab" are "Monoclonal AntiBodies".
ABO blood groups	Specific antigen system located on red blood cells (RBCs) and platelets (e.g. blood type A, B, AB or O). ABO blood type determination is an essential part of pre-transfusion testing for patients. Note: Patients with type A RBCs will have type B antibody in their plasma, while patients with type B RBCs will have type A antibody in their plasma. Since type O patient's red blood cells lack A antigen and B antigen, then not surprisingly they could have antibodies to both A and B antigens in their plasma. On the other hand, AB patients plasma is typically devoid of antibodies to either A or B antigen. Hence, the universal donor for RBCs is type O (devoid of A or B antigen) and universal donor for plasma is type AB (devoid of anti-A or Anti-B anti antibodies).
Acanthocyte	Also known as a spur cell, an acanthocyte is an RBC with irregular thorn-like projections. Looks like "cowboy boot spurs". These RBCs may be seen in some peripheral smears due to artifacts or may be associated with certain conditions including abetalipoproteinemia, liver disease, malnutrition, hypothyroidism, asplenia, and McLeod phenotype of Kell blood group, etc.
Acetylsalicylic acid	Also known as aspirin, it belongs to the non-steroid anti-inflammatory drug (NSAID) family which is used as an analgesic, antipyretic, and anti-inflammatory agent. Because of its anti-platelet properties, it is used in low dosage to prevent myocardial infarction, stroke, and thrombus formation. Main mechanism of actions includes irreversible binding of cyclooxygenase-1 (COX-1) and modification of Cox-2, thus decreases the production of prostaglandin and thromboxane A2. Hence, it irreversibly effects the function of the platelets and may be problematic if the patient is on aspirin and a surgical procedure is planned. Additionally, usage in children or adolescents for fever or other illnesses can cause Reye's syndrome.
Activated Partial Thromboplastin Time	Also known as aPTT or PTT, it is laboratory test that measures the integrity of the intrinsic pathway of coagulation and commonly used for monitoring heparin therapy. It is sensitive to detecting deficiencies in factors involved in the intrinsic pathway such as factor VIII, IX, XI, and XII common pathway such as factor X or phospholipid-dependent inhibitors such as lupus anticoagulants. As noted above, it is also prolonged if certain anticoagulants such as heparin are present. The test is performed by taking citrated plasma to clot at 37 degrees C after the addition of calcium (a set amount of phospholipid is also added but no Tissue Factor is added so it will not evaluate the extrinsic pathway). PTT could also be used comparatively in mixing studies when one suspects factor deficiency or presence of inhibitors. In a patient with a prolonged PTT (& normal PT), first the presence of heparin must be excluded. Once heparin is excluded, the patient's plasma can be mixed with a known normal plasma sample to see if the PTT corrects. Correction of the PTT in such setting is suggestive of a factor deficiency while lack of correction may imply presence of an inhibitor (antibody), such as lupus anticoagulant.
Activated-protein C resistance	APC resistance can be either acquired or inherited. The most common cause of APC resistance is due to a mutation at the cleavage site in Factor V, in which the amino acid Arg506 is replaced with Gln, producing Factor V Leiden. This mutation prevents APC from inactivating Factor V. APC resistance is usually associated with Factor V Leiden and results in an increased risk of thrombosis.

Acute	Generally refers to a process or disease that starts abruptly and/or progresses quickly. Examples include acute lymphoblastic leukemia (also known as ALL or acute lymphoblastic leukemia/lymphoma) & acute myeloid leukemia (AML) for neoplastic processes.
Acute lymphoblastic leukemia	Also known as ALL is an acute leukemia of lymphoid origin (B-cell origin is called B-ALL and T-cell origin is called T-ALL). Usually the peripheral blood, tissue and/or bone marrow shows an increase in number of lymphoblasts (typically greater than 20% in the peripheral blood and/or bone marrow as seen in many cases of B-ALL).
Acute myeloid leukemia	Acute leukemia of myeloid origin. Peripheral blood, tissue and/or bone marrow show increased number of myeloblasts (typically greater than 20% in the peripheral blood and/or bone marrow). Based on WHO 2008 criteria AMLs are divided into 1) AMLs with recurrent cytogenetic abnormalities (which typically have a better prognosis than the other AMLs) such as APL with t(15;17), AML with t(8;21), AML with t(16;16) or inv (16). 2) AML with Myelodysplasia-related changes (usually have a poor prognosis). 3) Therapy-Related AMLs (usually have a poor prognosis) and 4) AML-NOS which can be minimally differentiated, granulocytic origin (e.g. AML-M2), monocytic or myelomonocytic origin (AML-M4 & M5), erythroid origin (AML-M6) , or megakaryocytic origin (AML-M7). The prognosis on AML-NOS group is variable. Note: A blast with Auer rod(s) is by definition a myeloblast. Myeloblasts with Auer rod(s) have been noted in some AML-NOS (e.g. M2) and many times noted in APL.
Acute phase response	Is also known as acute phase reaction and is an inflammatory response to injury which may be related to an underlying infection, trauma, ischemia, immunologic or neoplastic process. During this reaction, the liver produces "acute phase proteins" which include but are not limited to CRP, fibrinogen, Factor VIII, ferritin, hepcidin, ceruloplasmin and haptoglobin. Hence, evaluating the levels of these proteins in the setting of inflammation may be problematic.
ADAMTS-13	A member of the metalloprotease family which is responsible for cleaving high molecular weight von Willebrand Factors (vWF). The cleavage of the vWF multimers reduces their size. Note: In thrombotic thrombocytopenic purpura (TTP) there is a decrease or absence of ADAMTS-13 which leads to larger vWF multimers that increases the chance of forming platelet thrombi and leading to microvascular thrombosis.
Adult T-cell Leukemia/Lymphoma	A systemic mature T-cell neoplasm that is associated with HTLV1 virus infection. Hence, this leukemia/lymphoma is more common in certain endemic areas such as parts of Japan, Africa and Caribbean islands.
Adverse hematologic reactions secondary to drugs	Adverse hematologic reactions to drugs include but are not limited to bone marrow suppression, agranulocytosis, thrombocytopenia, megaloblastoid changes, etc.
Afibrinogenemia	Afibrinogenemia and hypofibrinogenemia, refers to absence or reduction in the amount of the clotting factor fibrinogen in the blood. This is seen in rare instances as an inherited disorder, but more commonly it is seen with disseminated intravascular coagulation (DIC).

Agglutination	Aggregation or clumping of biologic substances such as bacteria or cells (e.g. red blood cell agglutination as noted in direct and indirect antiglobulin test, also known as Coombs' test). Agglutination may also be indicative of antibody-antigen presence on coated cells or substances.
Agranulocytosis	An adverse reaction that is usually due to certain drugs that leads to severe neutropenia and may be followed by fever and sore throat. Untreated, it may be deadly. Many drugs can cause agranulocytosis including but not limited to certain antibiotics, anti-thyroid medications, antihypertensive drugs, antipsychotic drugs, anti-inflammatory drugs, anticonvulsants, hypoglycemic drugs, and antidepressants.
AIHA	Autoimmune hemolytic anemia is usually due to autoantibodies (usually IgG) directed against RBCs. Hemolyic anemia results when splenic macrophages recognize the antibodies on the red cells resulting in phagocytosis and destruction. Some red cells escape complete destruction but loose membrane and surface area, resulting in circulating spherocytes.
Albumin	A major protein constituent of blood plasma. This protein is relatively negatively charged (as opposed to immunoglobulins which are relatively positively charged) and serves as a major protein in the plasma. It is produced in the liver so levels are usually reduced in end stage liver disease.
ALCL	Also known as anaplastic large cell lymphoma, it is usually an aggressive mature/maturing T-cell lymphoma that typically involve nodal tissue (e.g. lymph nodes) and sometimes skin (Cutaneous ALCL has better prognosis). The nodal ALCLs can be either ALK (Anaplastic Large cell Kinase) positive (better prognosis and a potential source of therapy) or ALK negative (worse prognosis in nodal ALCLs). Please note that the cutaneous ALCL is typically ALK negative with best prognosis. In summary: Amongst ALCLs, ALK negative cutaneous ALCL has the best prognosis while the Nodal ALK negative ALCL has the worst prognosis.
Alder-Reilly Anomaly	Evenly distributed violet purple granules without Döhle bodies or vacuoles in the cytoplasm of all neutrophils. Looks like toxic granules but unlike toxic granules, the findings are present in all the neutrophils and can also be seen in monocytes and lymphocytes. Please note that the granulocytes appear to be functionally normal. Hence, it is called an anomaly and not a disease.
Alemtuzumab	Also known as CAMPATH is a monoclonal antibody used in treating certain hematologic malignancies. Its mechanism of action is based on binding CD52 on cells and resulting in lysis. Note: Drugs ending with "MAB" are "Monoclonal AntiBodies".
Alkylating agents	A family of cytotoxic agents that are used in treatment of certain hematologic neoplasms. Their mechanism of action involves altering DNA and interfering with replication and transcription. Patients treated with these agents are at long term risk of developing other post treatment neoplastic disorders (e.g. myeloid disorders such as MDS and AML).
All-Trans Retinoic Acid	Also known as ATRA, it is an acid form of vitamin A, used to treat acute promyelocytic leukemia (APL).
Alloantibody	These are antibodies that recognizes non-self antigens. For example, alloantibodies can develop in patients who have received prior transfusions. Hence, having formed antibodies to non-self red blood cell antigens (e.g. anti-Kell, etc.). If a patient develops an alloantibody to Kell positive RBC, the next time this patient receives a Kell positive RBC transfusion, he or she may adversely react to the transfused blood and develop a hemolytic transfusion reaction which could be deadly. This is a major reason for testing a patient's blood prior to transfusing them with blood products.
Allogeneic	Typically refers to transferring tissue (e.g. bone marrow), blood, stem cells from one individual to another individual (e.g. allogeneic stem cell transplantation). The opposite of autologous which refers to being from self.

Alloimmunization	Formation of antibodies to non-self cellular antigens. Example includes formation of antibodies to non-self red blood cell antigens (e.g. anti-Kell, etc.).
Allopurinol	Brand name is Zyloprim. It is a purine analog drug used to treat hyperuricemia such as in the setting of gout. Rare but potentially fatal side effects include Stevens-Johnson syndrome (SJS) and toxic epidermal necrolysis (TEN). Can cause severe pancytopenia when used with azathioprine or mercaptopurine.
Allotype	It is usually a resultant of qualitative or quantitative difference in blood cell surface antigens between different individuals due to genetic polymorphism, ultimately leading to antigenic variation which can be recognized by alloantibodies.
Alpha granules	A type pf platelet granule. There are three types of granules present within platelets: alpha granules, delta (dense) granules and lysosomes. Alpha granules contain the larger molecules such as Platelet Factor 4 (PF4), Platelet-derived growth factor (PDGF), fibrinogen and some other clotting factors. The delta (dense) granules contain the smaller molecules such as serotonin, ADP, and calcium. Mnemonic is alpha stands for the "bigger" molecules such as proteins and peptides, while delta or dense stands for "diminutive" (tiny) molecules.
Alpha Storage Pool Disease	Also known as gray platelet syndrome, it is characterized by thrombocytopenia and abnormal enlarged gray-blue platelets with a washed-out appearance due to reduced alpha granules in platelets.
Alpha thalassemia	A type of thalassemia (Red blood cell disorder) that is specifically due to underproduction of the alpha hemoglobin chain, in contrast to beta thalassemia which is due to underproduction of beta hemoglobin chain. Note: As opposed to hemoglobinopathies which have intrinsic defects in the hemoglobin chain leading to abnormal hemoglobin molecules (e.g. sickle cell anemia), in thalassemias the hemoglobin molecule is usually not abnormal but rather underproduced.
Alpha-2-antiplasmin	A serine protease inhibitor that inactivates plasmin and fibrinolysis.
AML	Acute myeloid leukemia (AML) is an acute leukemia of myeloid origin. Peripheral blood, tissue and/or bone marrow show increased number of myeloblasts (typically greater than 20% in the peripheral blood and/or bone marrow). Based on WHO 2008 criteria AMLs are divided into 1) AMLs with recurrent cytogenetic abnormalities (which typically have a better prognosis than the other AMLs) such as APL with t(15;17), AML with t(8;21), AML with t(16;16) or inv (16). 2) AML with Myelodysplasia-related changes (usually have a poor prognosis). 3) Therapy-Related AMLs (usually have a poor prognosis) and 4) AML-NOS which can be minimally differentiated, granulocytic origin (e.g. AML-M2), monocytic or myelomonocytic origin (AML-M4 & M5), erythroid origin (AML-M6), or megakaryocytic origin (AML-M7). The prognosis on AML-NOS group is variable. Note: A blast with Auer rod(s) is by definition a myeloblast. Myeloblasts with Auer rod(s) have been noted in some AML-NOS (e.g. M2) and many times noted in APL.
Amyloidosis	A disease associated with deposition of amyloid in tissues. There are multiple different types of amyloids but the one typically seen in hematologic disorders is the AL (Amyloid Light chain) type which usually is associated with an underlying plasma cell neoplasm. The AL amyloid is associated with plasma cell neoplasms and are usually monoclonal light chains (kappa or lambda) leading to linear nonbranching fibril aggregates measuring 7.5-10 nm in width and ultimately comprised of beta-pleated sheets which can be highlighted with the congo red stain in tissue.
Anaplastic large cell lymphoma	Also known as ALCL, it is usually an aggressive mature/maturing T-cell lymphoma that typically involve nodal tissue (e.g. lymph nodes) and sometimes skin (cutaneous ALCL has better prognosis). The nodal ALCLs can be either ALK (Anaplastic Large cell Kinase) positive (better prognosis and a potential source of therapy) or ALK negative (worse prognosis in nodal ALCLs). Please note that the cutaneous ALCL is typically ALK negative with best prognosis. In summary: Amongst ALCLs, ALK negative cutaneous ALCL has the best prognosis while the nodal ALK negative ALCL has the worst prognosis.
Anemia	Refers to a decrease in hematocrit/hemoglobin levels (e.g. iron deficiency anemia). Anemias are typically classified into 3 broad categories: microcytic anemia (MCV <80), normocytic anemia (MCV 80-100), and macrocytic anemia (MCV > 100).
Angioimmunoblastic T-cell lymphoma	These are usually aggressive mature/maturing T-cell lymphomas that typically involve nodal tissue (lymph nodes). Patients with this lymphoma may have an underlying immune dysfunction and many are secondarily associated with EBV virus.

Anisocytosis	Refers to the variation in "size" of red blood cells. Laboratory value that correlates with anisocytosis is an elevated RDW.
Anti-D immunoglobulin	Antibody formed to one of the Rh antigens on red blood cells known as D antigen which can lead to red blood cell destruction. A classic example of this is seen in hemolytic disease of the newborn where the mother's anti-D antibodies attack and destroy the fetal Rh(D) positive red blood cells.
Anti-phospholipid syndrome	An autoimmune syndrome characterized by antibodies against phospholipids that causes thrombosis such as anti-cardiolipin antibodies, lupus anticoagulant antibodies, and anti-beta2 glycoprotein I antibodies. It is commonly associated with SLE and other autoimmune diseases. It can cause thrombosis and pregnancy-related complications such as preeclampsia and spontaneous abortion. Testing includes PTT, lupus anticoagulant antibody with dRVVT and testing for anticardiolipin.
Antibody	Also known as immunoglobulin, it is a protein that is produced by B cells (in terminally differentiated B-cells known as plasma cells these immunoglobulins are produced and secreted and are not cell surface bound) which recognize and bind to other proteins or substances (foreign or self antigens). Antibodies can be part of an immune response and help eradicate viruses and bacteria or may be part of an autoimmune destructive processes in hematology such as autoimmune hemolytic anemia or immune mediated platelet destruction (e.g. ITP).
Anticoagulant	These are natural or synthetic compounds that prevent the formation of blood clots. Common examples include heparin, warfarin (coumadin), etc.
Antigen	Typically refers to a molecular structure (on a foreign substance or self) which can be recognized by an antibody (e.g. foreign antigens include viral and bacterial components while self-antigens include certain aspects of a platelet or red blood cell, etc.).
APC resistance	Also known as activated-protein C resistance, this can be either acquired or inherited. The most common cause of APC resistance is due to a mutation at the cleavage site in Factor V, in which the amino acid Arg506 is replaced with Gln, producing Factor V Leiden. This mutation prevents APC from inactivating Factor V. APC resistance is usually associated with Factor V Leiden and results in an increased risk of thrombosis.
APL	Stands for acute promyelocytic leukemia. Usually has the following translocation, t(15;17) and is therefore responsive to ATRA therapy.

Aplastic anemia	A rare disorder that results in underproduction of bone marrow hematopoietic cells. Hence patients usually present with pancytopenia and their bone marrow appears markedly hypocellular.
Apoptosis	A form of cell death. As opposed to necrosis which is typically an abnormal process, apoptosis can be secondary to both normal and abnormal processes. Normal apoptosis is seen in lymph node germinal centers where the normal B-cells that are not selected undergo apoptosis. Abnormal processes with apoptosis include high grade lymphomas such as Burkitt lymphoma where there is a high rate of mitosis which leads to increased number of cells undergoing apoptosis.
Argatroban	Belongs to the class of univalent direct thrombin inhibitors, which also include Melagatran and Dabigatran. Called univalent because they bind only to the active site of the thrombin molecule. Used to treat Heparin-Induced Thrombocytopenia and can be monitored through PTT. It is cleared by the liver and therefore can be used in patients with renal insufficiencies.
Aspirin	Also known as acetylsalicylic acid, it belongs to the non-steroid anti-inflammatory drug (NSAID) family which is used as an analgesic, antipyretic, and anti-inflammatory agent. Because of its anti-platelet properties, it is used in low dosage to prevent myocardial infarction, stroke, and thrombus formation. Main mechanism of actions includes irreversible binding of cyclooxygenase-1 (COX-1) and modification of Cox-2, thus decreases the production of prostaglandin and thromboxane A2. Hence, it irreversibly effects the function of the platelets and may be problematic if the patient is on aspirin and planned for a surgical procedure. Additionally, usage in children or adolescents for fever or other illnesses can cause Reye's syndrome.
ATRA	Stands for All-Trans Retinoic Acid. It is the acid form of vitamin A which is used in treatment of acute promyelocytic leukemia (APL).
Auer rods	These are abnormal pink needle shaped polymerized granular structures found in the cytoplasm of abnormal myeloblasts that may be seen in certain myeloid neoplasms. Presence of Auer rods is typically associated with Acute myeloid leukemia (AML) and rarely associated with Refractory Anemia with Excess Blasts II (RAEB-II) which is the most aggressive type of MDS and usually progresses to AML.
Autoantibodies	These are antibodies that recognize self-antigens (e.g. autoimmune hemolytic anemia which can have autoantibodies, usually IgG, to RBCs and ultimately have the IgG-coated RBCs destroyed in the spleen, known as extravascular hemolysis).

Autologous	Typically refers to transferring tissue (e.g. bone marrow), blood, or stem cells from ones body to self (e.g. autologous stem cell transplantation).
B-ALL	Also known as B-cell lymphoblastic leukemia/lymphoma (or B-cell acute lymphoblastic leukemia), it is an acute leukemia of lymphoid origin (specifically B-cell origin). Usually the peripheral blood, tissue and/or bone marrow shows an increase in number of lymphoblasts (typically greater than 20% in the peripheral blood and/or bone marrow as seen in many cases of B-ALL).
B-cell	Type of white blood cell and more specifically a type of lymphocyte which produces antibodies (immunoglobulins). B-cells (like other hematopoietic cells) originate in the marrow and start maturation in the Bone marrow and complete their maturation process in germinal center of secondary follicles within secondary lymphoid tissues/organs such as lymph nodes, mucosa associated lymphoid tissue (MALT), or spleen. Remember B-cell for Bone marrow and T-cell for Thymus (B-cells start maturation in Bone marrow while T-cells mature in the Thymus.
Band	Refers to the band form of neutrophils. A maturing neutrophil that precedes the segmented neutrophils (PMNs) in the granulocytic maturation scheme. Increased numbers of Bands may be indicative of an underlying infection (especially bacterial).

Basophils	Type of white blood cell and more specifically granulocyte that maybe elevated in certain conditions such as but not limited to allergic reactions or CML.
Benign	Refers to a lesion or tumor that typically will not metastasize. The opposite of malignant.
Beta thalassemia	Beta thalassemia is due to underproduction of the beta hemoglobin chain. Due to underproduction of this beta chain, other globin chains such as the delta chain will compensate which is manifested by the increased level of Hemoglobin A2 (recall comprised of 2 alpha chains and 2 delta chains) noted in many of these patients.
Blast	Refers to an immature precursor of a white blood cell. Two types are myeloid (myeloblast) and lymphoid (lymphoblast).
Bleeding disorder	A disease that is typically due to clotting problems, either due to a defect or deficiency of platelets, platelet associated factors or clotting factors. Common examples include but are not limited to hemophilia A (Factor VIII deficiency), severe thrombocytopenia (e.g. platelet counts of less than 50 x 10^9/L).

Blood	Special fluid that is within vessels and is comprised of the cellular components (e.g. red blood cells, white blood cells and platelets) and plasma with proteins (e.g. clotting factors, vW factor, etc.).
Blood Bank	A section in most hospital's laboratory area which is responsible for collection, separation and storage of blood products such as red blood cells, platelets, fresh frozen plasma, etc.
Blood Smear	A glass slide prepared from peripheral blood for microscopic evaluation of the blood elements (e.g. red blood cells, white blood cells, platelets, etc.).
Bone marrow	The soft spongy cellular area in between the trabecular bony areas inside of the bone where blood's cellular components (e.g. red blood cells, white blood cells, and platelets) are produced.
Bone marrow serous fat atrophy	This usually refers to a hypocellular bone marrow with fat atrophy, and deposition of extracellular "gelatinous-like" material. This may be due to a damaged hematopoietic inductive microenvironment in the bone marrow and may be secondary to therapy (e.g. chemotherapy), HIV, or severe malnutrition.
Bone Marrow Transplant	Transfer of healthy bone marrow cells to an individual with diseased or damaged bone marrow.
Burkitt lymphoma	An aggressive mature/maturing B-cell lymphoma which is characterized by intermediate-sized cells with a very high mitotic index (Ki67 close to 100%). The typical immunophenotype is CD19+, CD20+, CD10+, CD5-, and BCL2-. The classic translocation associated with this lymphoma is the t(8;14) which involves c-MYC and IgH (see lymphoma mnemonic diagram below for an easy way to remember this and other common B-cell lymphomas).
Cancer	An abnormal growth of malignant cells with a chance of spreading (metastasis) to other sites.

Castleman disease	A heterogenous group of diseases that present with lymphadenopathy with variable presentations and prognosis. There are 3 main types: 1) Hyaline vascular variant (most common subtype, more common in younger patients, usually asymptomatic, localized disease, and best prognosis); 2) Plasma cell variant (many are localized and more common in elderly with systemic symptoms such as anemia, thrombocytopenia, elevated ESR, elevated IL6, and polyclonal hypergammaglobulinemia); 3) Multicentric variant (some similarities to the plasma cell variant with similar systemic symptoms and more common in elderly). However, this variant as the name implies usually involves multiple lymph nodes, is often seen in HIV positive patients, usually HHV8 positive, and has the worst prognosis. Additionally, it can be also associated with other HHV8 positive neoplasms such Kaposi sarcoma.
CBC	Complete Blood Count which includes a count of the WBC, hemoglobin, hematocrit and platelets. When a differential count is added to the CBC, the different types of WBCs are quantitated (e.g. percent neutrophils, lymphocytes, monocytes, eosinophils and basophils).
CD	Stands for "Cluster of Differentiation" which are usually cell surface glycoproteins expressed by normal and abnormal cells and used in diagnostic hematology as part of the workup by either flow cytometry or immunohistochemistry (e.g. co-expression of CD5 and CD23 by the neoplastic cells in CLL).
CD mnemonic	The mnemonic is "T" for "Tiny" CDs and "T-cells" referring to the fact that typically the Tiny CDs (CD1, 2, 3, 4, 5, 6, 7, & 8) are expressed in T-cells as opposed to "B" for "B-cells" & "Bigger" CDs (CD19, 20, 21, 22, 23, and 24) which are typically expressed in "B-cells". The "Middle" CDs (CD11, 12, 13, 14, 15, 16, 17 & 18) are more commonly expressed in "MyeloMonocytic" (M for Middle and M for Myelomonocytic referring to granulocytes and monocytes). Note: The above mnemonic is mainly for the normal T-cells, Myeloid cells and B-cells. Abberant expression may be seen in other lineages in diseased states and some common examples include the expression of the T-cell marker CD7 on abnormal myeloblasts in some AMLs or the abnormal expression of the T-cell marker CD5 on CLL or Mantle Cell Lymphoma.
CD1a	A type of CD which is normally expressed in immature thymic T-cells (e.g. cortical thymocytes) and dendritic cells. Also remember that since this is the lowest numbered CD, then it is typically only expressed in immature T-cells (cortical thymocytes) and not present in more mature T-cells.
CD2	A type of CD which is normally expressed in most T-cells (immature and mature).
CD3	A type of CD which is normally expressed in most T-cells (immature and mature). CD3 is the most specific T-cell marker.
CD4	A type of CD which is normally expressed in a subset of T-cells (Helper T-cells). This CD is also expressed in lower levels on monocytes. Also recall the rule of 8 mnemonic: CD4 associates with MCH Class II (4x2 =8), while CD8 associates with MHC Class I (8x1=8).
CD5	A type of CD which is normally expressed in most T-cells (immature and mature). CD5 can also be seen in very small subset of normal B-cells and also aberrantly (abnormally) expressed in certain B-cell lymphoma/leukemias (e.g. CLL and Mantle cell Lymphoma).
CD7	A type of CD which is normally expressed in most T-cells (immature and mature). This is the earliest expressed CD T-cell marker.
CD8	A type of CD which is normally expressed in a subset of T-cells (Cytotoxic T-cells). This CD is can also be expressed in lower levels on some NK-cells. Also recall the rule of 8 mnemonic: CD4 associates with MCH Class II (4x2 =8), whereas CD8 associates with MHC Class I (8x1=8).
CD10	A CD that can be seen expressed in a variety of cell types (hematopoietic and non-hematopoietic). In hematopoietic cells CD10 is commonly expressed in mature neutrophils, early B-cells (hematogones), germinal center B-cells, and certain germinal center derived malignancies, such as follicular lymphoma.
CD11b	Commonly expressed on myelomonocytic cells including granulocytes, monocytes and some AMLs.

CD13	Commonly expressed on myelomonocytic cells including granulocytes, monocytes (brighter expression), and many AMLs. Remember from the CD Mnemonic, "M" for Middle CDs (CD11 through CD18) and "M" for MyeloMonocytic cells.
CD14	A CD that is expressed on mature or maturing monocytes. Remember from the CD Mnemonic, "M" for Middle CDs (CD11 through CD18) and "M" for MyeloMonocytic cells.
CD15	Commonly expressed on maturing myelomonocytic cells including granulocytes, monocytes and some AMLs. Remember from the CD Mnemonic, "M" for Middle CDs (CD11 through CD18) and "M" for MyeloMonocytic cells.
CD16	Commonly expressed on maturing myelomonocytic cells including granulocytes, monocytes and some AMLs. Remember from the CD Mnemonic, "M" for Middle CDs (CD11 through CD18) and "M" for MyeloMonocytic cells.
CD19	A type of CD which is normally expressed in most B-cells including normal plasma cells. Recall the CD Mnemonic, "B" for "B-cells" & "Bigger" CDs (CD19, 20, 21, 22, 23, 24) which are typicaly expressed in "B-cells". Most B-cell lymphoma/leukemias are CD19 positive. In contrast to normal plasma cells which express CD19, most plasma cell neoplasms (e.g. Plasma Cell Myeloma) do not express CD19.
CD20	A type of CD which is normally expressed in most mature B-cells. It is usually negative in early hematogones and normal plasma cells. Recall the CD Mnemonic, "B" for "B-cells" & "Bigger" CDs (CD19, 20, 21, 22, 23, 24) which are typicaly expressed in "B-cells". Most mature B-cell lymphoma/leukemias are CD20 positive. CD20 is typically negative in most plasma cell neoplasms (e.g. plasma cell myeloma). CD20 expression on lymphomas is also very important clinically since there is an anti-CD20 drug (Rituximab) that is typically used as part of the treatment of these lymphomas.
CD21	Expressed on B-cells and follicular dendritic cells. Co-receptor for Epstein Barr Virus (EBV) which explains why B-cells are typically the cells infected by EBV and not T-cells (T-cells lack CD21). Recall the CD Mnemonic, "B" for "B-cells" & "Bigger" CDs (CD19, 20, 21, 22, 23, 24) which are typicaly expressed in "B-cells". Note: Unfortunately the function and expression profile of CDs larger than CD24 need to be memorized.
CD22	A CD which is normally expressed in most B-cells (both immature and mature) but not typically expressed in plasma cells. Recall the CD Mnemonic, "B" for "B-cells" & "Bigger" CDs (CD19, 20, 21, 22, 23, 24) which are typicaly expressed in "B-cells". Note: Unfortunately the function and expression profile of CDs larger than CD24 need to be memorized.
CD23	Expressed on B-cells and follicular dendritic cells. Recall the CD Mnemonic, "B" for "B-cells" & "Bigger" CDs (CD19, 20, 21, 22, 23, 24) which are typicaly expressed in "B-cells". Note: Unfortunately the function and expression profile of CDs larger than CD24 need to be memorized.
Chediak-Higashi syndrome	Autosomal recessive disorder leading to a microtubule polymerization defect that reduces phagolysosome formation and phagocytic activity. Hence reduced bacteriacidal function. It is characterized by albinism, peripheral neuropathy and increased risk of pyogenic infections. Characteristic neutrophils with chunky large granules.
Chemotherapy	A medical treatment used in destroying cancer cells.
Chronic	A slow growing or progressing process. The opposite of acute. (e.g. chronic lymphocytic leukemia or chronic inflammation).

Chronic lymphocytic leukemia	Also known as CLL. An indolent B-cell leukemia more common in the elderly population. Characteristic immunophenotype (dim CD20+, CD19+, CD5+, CD23+, CD10- monotypic dim kappa or dim lambda B-cells). The disease has two forms: CLL if it is in the blood (hence, "leukemia") and SLL (small lymphocytic lymphoma) if it is in the tissue such as lymph nodes (hence, "Lymphoma"). Mnemonic: As opposed to acute lymphoblastic leukemia (ALL) which are "immature" cells and more common in "pediatric" (less mature) population, CLL is comprised of "mature" lymphocytes and predominantly seen in the elderly (more mature) population. 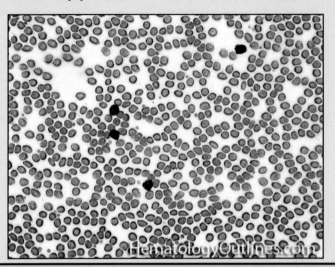
Chronic myelogenous leukemia	Also known as CML, this is a myeloproliferative neoplasm of abnormal bone marrow stem cells that is characterized by the chromosome translocation t(9;22) which leads to a BCR-ABL1 fusion gene (Philadelphia chromosome). Initially presents as an indolent chronic phase with subsequent transition to accelerated phase and sometimes blast phase. First line therapy usually includes "Imatinib" (also known as Gleevec). Similar to most of the other myeloproliferative neoplasms, patients usually present with some elevated count or "cytosis" (such as elevated WBC count which is known as leukocytosis) and splenomegaly. The peripheral blood smear usually shows leukocytosis with increased number of myeloid (granulocytic) precursors in different phases of maturation (Clue: the peripheral blood smear looks like a bone marrow aspirate smear). 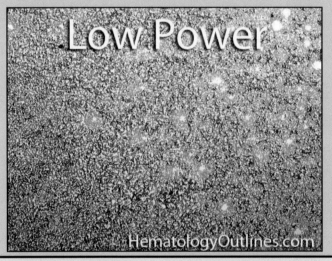
Chronic Myelomonocytic Leukemia	Also known as CMML, this is an abnormal bone marrow stem cell disorder that has characteristic features of both a myeloproliferative neoplasm ("cytosis" specifically monocytosis and splenomegaly) and a myelodysplastic syndrome (dysplastic cells). Hence, per WHO 2008 criteria, it belongs to the category of myeloproliferative/myelodysplastic disorders. At the time of diagnosis, they usually present with leukocytosis and history of a "persistent monocytosis" is typically required. In contrast to CML, there is no BCR-ABL1 fusion.

CLL	Also known as chronic lymphocytic leukemia. An indolent B-cell leukemia more common in elderly population. Characteristic immunophenotype (dim CD20+, CD19+, CD5+, CD23+, CD10- monotypic dim kappa or dim lambda B-cells). The disease has two forms: CLL if it is in the blood (hence, "leukemia") and SLL (small lymphocytic lymphoma) if it is in the tissue such as lymph nodes (hence, "Lymphoma"). Mnemonic: As opposed to acute lymphoblastic leukemia (ALL) which are "immature" cells and more common in "pediatric" (less mature) population, CLL is comprised of "mature" lymphocytes and predominantly seen in elderly (more mature) population.
Clot	Usually refers to "blood clot" (also known as thrombus). The final product of coagulation pathway in hemostasis (platelets and coagulation factors). Normally formed at the site of injury. If exaggerated, it may lead to thrombosis (pathologic). Recall Virchow's Triad which increase risk of thrombosis: 1) Hypercoagulability (e.g. Cancer patients), 2) Abnormal blood flow (e.g.due to stasis), & 3) Endothelial injury (e.g.post trauma).
Clotting factors	Proteins within blood plasma involved in the formation and stabalization of the blood clot. Common examples include factors I, II, V, VII, VIII, IX, X, and XI.
Cluster of Differentiation	Also known as "CD". These are glycoproteins expressed by normal and abnormal cells and can be used as part of the diagnostic workup in many hematologic malignancies by either flow cytometry or immunohistochemistry (e.g. co-expression of CD5 and CD23 on CLL cells).
CMML	Also known as chronic myelomonocytic leukemia, it is an abnormal bone marrow stem cell disorder that has characteristic features of both a myeloproliferative neoplasm ("cytosis" specifically Monocytosis and splenomegaly) and a Myelodysplastic syndrome (dysplastic cells). Hence, per WHO 2008 criteria, it belongs to the category of myeloproliferative/myelodysplastic disorders. At the time of diagnosis, they usually present with leukocytosis and history of a "persistent monocytosis" is typically required. As opposed to CML, there is no BCR-ABL1 fusion.

Coagulopathy	This usually refers to a bleeding or clotting disorder which is typically secondary to an impairment of the blood's ability to form a thrombus (clot). Mostly the defect or deficiency of the coagulation factors leads to an increased risk of bleed (e.g. Hemophilia A due to factor VIII deficiency or vW disease due to a defect or deficiency of vW factor) but sometimes the deficiency may lead to an increased risk of thrombosis (clottting) such as in Factor XII deficiency.
Cold agglutinins	Usually associated with a cold-reacting IgM antibody that is usually not clinically significant at body temperature. On peripheral smear you may see RBC agglutination (Clumping of RBCs). However, cold agglutinins may cause cold agglutinin disease.
Complete Blood Count	Also known as CBC which includes a count of the WBC, hemoglobin, hematocrit and platelets. When a differential count is added to the CBC, the different types of WBCs are quantitated (e.g. percent neutrophils, lymphocytes, monocytes, eosinophils and basophils).
Coombs test	Also known as an antiglobulin test. There are two types: Direct Antiglobulin Test (DAT) and Indirect Antiglobulin Test (IAT). Direct detects Abs or complement bound to patient's RBCs while Indirect detects Abs against RBCs in the patient's Serum (plasma). An example of DAT positive disease is autoimmune hemolytic anemia. An example of IAT is detecting alloantibodies in the patient's plasma prior to transfusing them with a specific type of RBC (e.g. Kell negative RBC).
Coumadin	Generic name: Warfarin is an anticoagulant that acts by inhibiting the vitamin K-dependent synthesis of factors II, VII, IX, and X, as well as proteins C & S. Used in the prevention of thrombosis and clinical settings such as atrial fibrillation, the presence of artificial heart valves, deep venous thrombosis, and pulmonary embolism. Degree of anticoagulation is monitored by INR. Coumadin is contraindicated in pregnancy. Adverse effects include hemorrhage, warfarin necrosis, and osteoporosis. Effects of Coumadin can be reversed by giving vitamin K. Fresh-frozen plasma (FFP) can be given when rapid reversal is needed.
D-Dimer	Products of a blood clot degeneration or breakdown. Can be the result of plasmin degrading fibrin into D-dimer (two cross-linked D fragments of the fibrinogen protein). Hence it is a type of FDP. Usually increased after thrombotic events and Disseminated Intravascular Coagulation (DIC). Note: D-Dimer levels can be used to exclude thrombosis if the probability of thrombosis is low and the D-Dimer is negative (good negative predictive value).
Delta granules	Also known as dense bodies, these are secretory organelles in platelets containing ADP, ATP, calcium and serotonin. Compared to alpha granules, these are all smaller molecules. Mnemonic is "Delta or Dense" granules are Diminutive (tiny molecules) as opposed to alpha granules.
Deoxyhemoglobin	Hemoglobin that is not bound to oxygen (oxygenated hemoglobin unloads oxygen in tissue and becomes deoxyhemoglobin).
DIC	Disseminated Intravascular Coagulation is a microangiopathic hemolytic anemia that is characterized by thrombocytopenia and consumption of coagulation factors (i.e. there is usually an increase in both PT and PTT lab tests). DIC is not a disease by itself but rather secondary to an underlying disease process (e.g. secondary to infection, malignancy, trauma, etc.). On peripheral smears, one may see increased numbers of schistocytes which are caused by fibrin-induced intravascular hemolysis.

Disseminated Intravascular Coagulation	Also known as DIC, it is a microangiopathic hemolytic anemia that is characterized by thrombocytopenia and consumption of coagulation factors (i.e. there is usually an increase in both PT and PTT lab tests). DIC is not a disease by itself but rather secondary to an underlying disease process (e.g. secondary to infection, malignancy, trauma, etc.). On peripheral smears one may see increased numbers of schistocytes which may have been caused by a fibrin-induced intravascular hemolysis.
Döhle bodies	Blue-gray cytoplasmic inclusions (remnants of rough ER) that may be seen in neutrophils. Increased numbers may be indicative of an underlying inflammatory condition and/or infection. If döhle bodies are accompanied by giant platelets, it may be due to May Hegglin anomaly.
dRVVT	Also known as Dilute Russell Viper Venom Time, it is an in vitro qualitative test for lupus anticoagulant (LA) and usually follows an elevated PTT when LA is suspected. The test is derived from the venom of Russell viper, a power thrombotic agent in vitro. A mixing study is performed combining Russell viper venom, patient's plasma, and phospholipids, which is required for coagulation. The presence of Lupus Anticoagulant would prevent clotting. A prolonged clotting time would be followed up with a confirmatory test where excess phospholipids are added to the mixing study, which should overcome LA and induce clotting. A ratio between clotting time without excess phospholipids and with excess phospholids is then calculated. An elevated ratio is considered positive and consistent with LA.
Dutcher bodies	Intranuclear pseudoinclusions noted in plasma cells. Usually associated with abnormal plasma cells such as plasmacytoma or plasma cell myeloma.
Dys	Dys means abnormal. Examples include dyserythropoiesis (abnormal erythroid maturation), dysplasia (abnormal growth or abnormal formation), etc.
EBV	Epstein Barr Virus. A virus associated with infectious mononucleosis (a disease more common in younger patients that presents with lymphadenopathy and in severe cases with organomagly such as hepatomegaly and/or Splenomegaly). EBV may also be associated with certain lymphoproliferative disorders such as post transplant lymphoproliferative disorders (PTLD), angioimmunoblastic T-cell lymphoma and Hodgkin lymphoma.
Eculizumab	Brand name: Soliris. It is a recombinant monoclonal antibody directed against complement protein C5. It inhibits the cleavage of C5 by C5 convertase which prevents the generation of the membrane attack complex, C5b-C9. Eculizumab is used to treat paroxysmal nocturnal hemoglobinuria (PNH) which is a disease characterized by complement-mediate intravascular hemolysis. This drug has also been used to treat certain Hemolytic Uremic Syndrome (HUS) cases.

Elliptocytes	Oval shaped RBCs (also known as ovalocytes). These can be seen in variety of conditions including iron deficiency anemia and hereditary elliptocytosis. 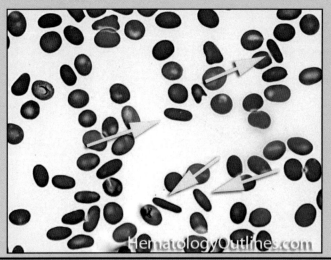
Eosinophils	A type of WBC seen in peripheral blood and tissue. It belongs to the myeloid lineage and more specifically a subtype of granulocyte with bright eosinophilic (red) granules containing Major Basic Protein, histamine, and plasminogen. Increased numbers of eosinophils in blood can be due to many things (remember the major classes for most differential diagnosis include an underlying infection, malignancy, autoimmune, trauma, congenital, drug-induced or idiopathic). Increased eosinophils may be due to an infection (e.g. tissue invasive parasites), malignancy (e.g. Hodgkin lymphoma, carcinoma or chronic eosinophilic leukemia), autoimmune, drug-induced (e.g. certain antibiotics, etc.), or idiopathic causes. 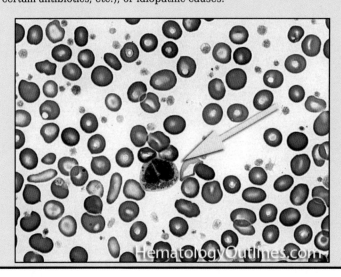

172

Eosinophilia	Refers to an increased number of eosinophils in the blood. DDx: Secondary to a tissue invasive parasitic infection, autoimmune, malignancy, drugs, or idiopathic causes).
EPO	Also known as erythropoietin, it is a glycoprotein hormone that stimulates erythropoiesis. It is mainly produced by the liver during the fetal period and by the kidney in adults. Manufactured EPO is typically used to treat anemia due to chronic renal disease, myelodysplasia, and anemia associated with cancer treatment (post chemotherapy and radiation).
Erythrocyte	Another name for Red Blood Cell (RBC). Belongs to the myeloid cell lineage. RBCs main role is to carry and deliver oxygen through hemoglobin.
Erythroid maturation	Erythroids (RBCs) start as nucleated cells in the marrow and ultimately lose their nucleus prior to leaving the marrow and entering the blood.
Erythrophagocytosis	Refers to RBCs ingested (phagocytosed) by macrophages and sometimes other WBCs.

Erythropoietin	Also known as EPO, it is a glycoprotein hormone that stimulates erythropoiesis. It is mainly produced by the liver during the fetal period and by the kidney in adults. Manufactured EPO is typically used to treat anemia due to chronic renal disease, myelodysplasia, and anemia associated with cancer treatment (post chemotherapy and radiation).
FAB classification	FAB stands for French, American, British which was the old classification scheme used in classifying certain hematologic malignancies such as Acute Myeloid Leukemias (AMLs M0 through M7), Acute Lymphoblastic Leukemia (ALL) and Myelodysplastic Syndromes (MDS).
Faggot cell	Collection of Auer rods sometimes seen within blasts (also called a faggot cell, which means "bundle of sticks") in Acute Promyelocytic Leukemia (APL).
FDP	Fibrin degradation products (FDP) are the result of blood clot degeneration or breakdown. Can be the result of plasmin degrading fibrin into FDPs (e.g. D-Dimer which is a type of FDP: Two Cross-linked D fragments of fibrinogen protein). FDPs are increased after thrombotic events and Disseminated Intravascular Coagulation (DIC). Note: D-Dimer (a type of FDP) levels can be used to exclude thromobosis if the probability of thrombosis is low and the D-Dimer is negative.
Ferritin	A protein that is present in many cell types and serves to store Iron. It is also an Acute Phase Protein meaning that it's levels may rise in a background of inflammation or stress.
Fibrin degradation product	Also known as FDP are products of a blood clot degeneration. Can be the result of plasmin degrading fibrin into FDPs (e.g. D-Dimer: Two Cross-linked D fragments of fibrinogen protein). FDPs are increased after thrombotic events and Disseminated Intravascular Coagulation (DIC). Note: D-Dimer (a type of FDP) levels can be used to exclude thromobosis if the probability of thrombosis is low and the D-Dimer is negative.
Fibrinogen	Also known as Factor I, it is a glycoprotein synthesized in the liver that is involved in coagulation cascade. Fibrinogen is cleaved by thrombin to form fibrin. Fibrin is then cross-linked by Factor XIII to form a clot. Note: Fibrinogen is also an acute-phase reactant which is elevated during inflammation.
Flow cytometry	A laboratory test that characterizes cells based on their immunophenotype by using antibodies that tag cell surface or nuclear epitopes. It is analogous to the concept of tissue immunohistochemistry (IHC). Advantages of flow cytometry over IHC are: quicker turn-around time, being able to evaluate multiple antibodies on a cell population simultaneously, etc. It is commonly used in diagnostic hematology to characterize hematologic malignancies (Acute Leukemias, Lymphomas, etc.).
Fludarabine	Brand name: Fludara. It is a chemotherapy drug used to treat chronic lymphocytic leukemia (CLL), salvage therapy of non-Hodgkin lymphoma, and acute myeloid leukemias (AML). Side effects include anemia, thrombocytopenia, neutropenia, and profound lymphopenia.
Folate Deficiency	Folate, also known as folic acid, is a water-soluble vitamin with an important role in DNA synthesis and repair. It is typically given during pregnancy to prevent neural tube defects in the embryo. Deficiency in folate or folic acid can also result in macrocytic anemia. Methotrexate, a drug that interferes with folate metabolism, inhibits the production of tetrahydrofolate (THF), an active form of folic acid, and can cause inflammation in the GI tract and marrow suppression. Therefore, folate supplement is usually given to reverse the toxic side effects of methotrexate. Folic acid, together with vitamin B12, is important in the conversion of homocysteine to methionine, therefore folate and/or vitamin B12 deficiency can lead to hyperhomocyteinemia (see vitamin B12). However, as opposed to B12 deficiency, MMA is not elevated in Folate deficiency since it is not involved in the conversion of methylmalonyl-CoA to succinyl-CoA in the Kreb cycle. Take home points: Folate deficiency may show hyperhomocyteinemia but no elevation in MMA (Methyl Malonic Acid). While B12 deficiency may show both hyperhomocyteinemia and an elevated MMA.

Follicular lymphoma	A common mature B-cell lymphoma that usually shows a nodular growth pattern and more commonly behaves in a low grade fashion. Immunophenotypically the neoplastic B-cells in this lymphoma are CD19+ and CD20+ ("Big" CDs meaning "B" cell origin), CD10+ and BCL2+. The common translocation associated with this lymphoma is t(14;18) which includes IgH and BCL2 genes, see Lymphoma mnemonic. 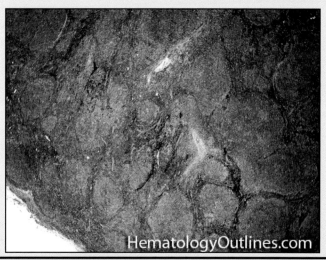
Fragmented red blood cells	Also known as schistocytes and helmet cells, these are irregularly shaped assymetrical fragments of RBCs that may have several morphologic forms. It is usually the result of mechanical disruption of the RBCs. They can be generated by getting stuck to fibrin strands within the vasculature secondary to an underlying Microangiopathic hemolytic anemia such as HUS, TTP and DIC or broken up by a mechanical heart valve. 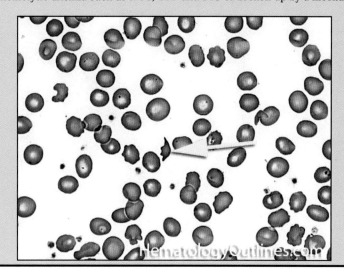

G6PD deficiency	An enzyme deficiency that makes RBCs more susceptible to oxidative damage. This oxidative damage is in the hemoglobin molecules which precipitates out as Heinz bodies which are then deposited on RBC membrane and can be phagocytized by splenic macrophages leading to bite cells (RBCs that look like someone has taken a bite out of them). Conditions that may increase the chance of oxidative damage in these patients include infections, certain sulfa drugs, or fava beans.
	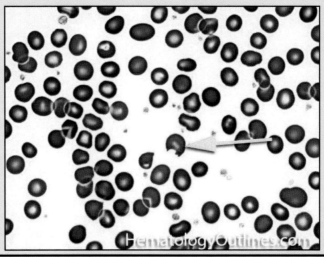
GCSF	Generic name: Filgrastim, Brand name: Neupogen. It is a granulocyte colony-stimulating factor, a growth factor hormone that stimulates the bone marrow to produce granulocytes and stem cells. It is used to accelerate recovery from neutropenia after chemotherapy and as a supportive medication used to prevent infection and neutropenic fevers. GCSF is also used to increase the number of hematopoietic stem cells in the blood of donors before collection by leukopheresis for use in hematopoietic stem cell transplantation.
Germinal center	These are the central portion of the secondary follicles in lymphoid tissue (e.g. lymph node, MALT, or spleen). As the primary follicle (no germinal center) gets antigen stimulated, the primary follicle then turns into a secondary follicle (germinal center is in the middle of these secondary follicles). Upon antigen stimulation, B-cells within these germinal centers continue their maturation cycle by undergoing somatic hypermuatation and heavy chain class switching which could ultimately lead to the development of a plasma cell or memory B-cell.
	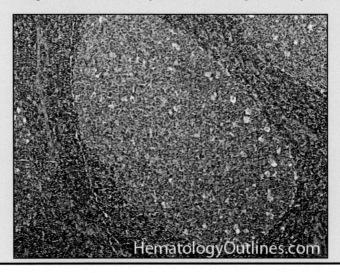

Giant platelets	Very large platelets. Usually equal to or larger than the size of a normal RBC. Increased numbers in peripheral blood smears may be indicative of an underlying marrow or myeloid disorder.
	 HematologyOutlines.com
Globin chain	This usually refers to one of the peptide chains that comprise the hemoglobin molecule. There are multiple types of globin chains with various combinations that comprise different hemoglobin molecules. These include the alpha, beta, gamma and delta chains. Combination of these globin chains gives rise to multiple types of normal hemoglobin molecules. In order of most to least prevalent Hemoglobins, Hemoglobin A (HbA) is comprised of 2 Alphas + 2 Beta chains, Hemoglobin A2 (HbA2) is comprised of 2 Alphas + 2 Delta chains, and Hemoglobin F (HbF) is comprised of 2 Alphas + 2 Gamma chains.
Glucocorticoids	A class of steroid hormones produced by the adrenal cortex and involved in immune regulation and glucose metabolism by acting through glucocorticoid receptors. An example is cortisol, produced by the zona fasiculata in the adrenal cortex, which regulates blood sugar through gluconeogenesis, suppresses the immune system, and aids in fat, protein and carbohydrate metabolism. Synthetic form is manufactured and used to replace physiologic deficits, such as in adrenal insufficiencies, produce therapeutic immunosuppression, and as anti-inflammatory modulators.
Granulation tissue	A reparative process in tissues that is usually post-injury. Eventually, the goal of the injured tissue is to form a granulation tissue and ultimately recruit fibroblasts and lead to fibrosis. Not to be confused with granuloma (granulomatous inflammation) which by definition is a collection of epithelioid histiocytes.
Granulocytes	Belongs to the myeloid lineage. There are three different types: Neutrophils (with neutral staining granules), Eosinophils (with Eosinophilic or red staining granules), and Basophils (with basophilic or blue/purple staining granules).
	 HematologyOutlines.com

Granuloma	Also known as granulomatous inflammation, it is a collection of epithelioid histiocytes (large histiocytes with increased cytoplasm). May be due to an underlying infection (e.g. Mycobacterial or fungi), Malignancy (e.g. Hodgkin Lymphoma), or other processes (e.g. Sarcoidosis). Not to be confused with granulation tissue.
Granulomatous Inflammation	Also known as granuloma, it is a collection of epithelioid histiocytes (large histiocytes with increased cytoplasm). May be due to an underlying infection (e.g. Mycobacterial or fungi), malignancy (e.g. Hodgkin lymphoma), or other processes (e.g. sarcoidosis). Not to be confused with granulation tissue.
Gray platelet syndrome	Also known as Alpha Granule Deficiency, it is a rare inherited bleeding disease that is due to loss of alpha granules in platelets. Recall, alpha granules contain the larger molecules such as PDGF, PF-4, Fibronectin and vWF (as opposed to delta or dense granules that contain the smaller molecules such as serotonin, ADP, ATP and Calcium).
H bodies	Also known as Hemoglobin H, it is an abnormal hemoglobin (Beta chain tetramer) that is the result of excess B-chain production due to underproduction of alpha chains in severe alpha thalassemia.
Hairy cell leukemia	An indolent B-cell leukemia with leukemic cells (abnormal cells circulating in the blood) that have cytoplasmic projections resembling "Hair-like" projections. Patients usually present with some cytopenia and splenomegaly with the neoplastic cells involving the red pulp of the spleen. The typical immunophenotype of hairy cell is CD19+, CD20+, CD25+, CD103+ and CD11c+.

Haptoglobin	A serum protein that can bind free hemoglobin. Hence, after intravascular hemolysis, the free haptoglobin binds the released hemoglobin molecules so the levels of the measured free haptoglobin will fall. Note: A low haptoglobin lab value could be secondary to an intravascular hemolysis or sometimes due to severe extravascular hemolysis.
Hb	Abbreviation of hemoglobin. A major protein in Red blood cells (RBCs) that is responsible for carrying oxygen. It is composed of four peptide chains. The three major normal hemoglobins are Hb-A (2 alpha chains and 2 Beta chains), Hb-A2 (2 alpha chains and 2 delta chains), and Hb-F (2 alpha chains and 2 gamma chains). Hemoglobin can be measured along with Hct, WBC and platelets as part of a routine CBC (complete blood count). Decreased hemoglobin and Hct levels are indicative of anemia.
Hct	Abbreviation of hematocrit. A percentage of blood that is taken up by RBCs. Low levels is usually indicative of anemia. The normal ratio of hemoglobin to hematocrit is about 1:3 (e.g. hemoglobin of 10 g/dL usually coorelates with a Hematocrit of 30%).
Heinz bodies	Abnormal precipitated hemoglobins usually due to oxidative damage. These may be seen in conditions that predispose a patient's hemoglobin to oxidative damage (e.g. G6PD deficiency). Remember "HEinz" start with HE which stands for HEmoglobin (as opposed to Howell-Jolly Bodies which are DNA remnants).
Helmet cell	Also known as schistocyte, it is an irregularly shaped asymmetrical fragment of RBC that may have several morphologic forms. It is usually the result of mechanical disruption of the RBCs. They can be generated by getting stuck to fibrin strands within the vasculature secondary to an underlying microangiopathic hemolytic anemia such as HUS, TTP and DIC or broken up by a mechanical heart valve.
Helper T cell	These are a type of T-cell lymphocyte that express CD4 and do not have cytotoxic or phagocytic capabilities. Increased numbers of CD4+ T-cells could be due to a maligancy such as T-cell lymphoma (neoplastic T-cells) or Hodgkin lymphoma (non-neoplastic background T-cells), certain infections such as Mycobacterium tuberculosis or fungi with granulomatous inflammation (granuloma).

Hematocrit	Also known as Hct. A percentage of blood that is taken up by RBCs. Low levels is usually indicative of anemia. The normal ratio of hemoglobin to hematocrit is about 1:3 (e.g. Hemoglobin of 10 g/dL usually coorelates with a Hematocrit of 30%).
Hematogones	Early B-cells in the developmental stage following precursor B-cells and before small naïve B-cell found in the bone marrow. Hematogones are more abundant in normal infant marrow and less common in normal adult marrow. A normal hematogone population shows a range of morphology and immunophenotype reflecting a spectrum of maturation. The typical morphology of hematogones is CD19+ and CD10+ with variable expression of CD34, TdT and CD20 depending on their maturation stage. They typically do not express Kappa or Lambda light chains. 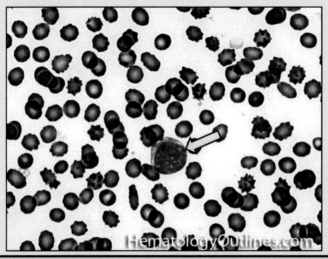
Hematopoietic cells	These are bone marrow cells that include myeloid (Granulocytic, Monocytic, Erythroid, and megakaryocytic lineages) and lymphoid (T-cell, B-cell, and Nk-cell) cells. 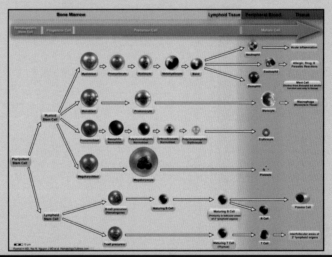
Heme	Consists of iron in the center of a porphyrin ring. Heme is a constituent of certain oxygen binding molecules such as hemoglobin or myoglobin and in its normal state its iron is in the ferrous state (Fe++). When oxidized, the Fe++ (hemoglobin) becomes Fe+++ (methemoglobin). An example of this is noted in bleeding patients when their bright red blood (Fe++) is exposed to outside air and oxidized forming a dark brown color (Fe+++).
Hemoglobin	Abbreviated as Hb. A major protein in Red blood cells (RBCs) that is responsible for carrying oxygen. It is composed of four peptide chains. The three major normal hemoglobins are Hb-A (2 alpha chains and 2 Beta chains), Hb-A2 (2 alpha chains and 2 delta chains), and Hb-F (2 alpha chains and 2 gamma chains). The Hemoglobin value can be measured along with Hct, WBC and platelets as part of a routine CBC. Decreased hemoglobin and Hct levels are indicative of anemia. The normal ratio of hemoglobin to hematocrit is about 1:3 (e.g. Hemoglobin of 10 g/dL usually correlates with a Hematocrit of 30%).

Hemoglobin C disease	A hemoglobinopathy that is due to a mutation that changes a hydrophilic residue (glutamate) on the hemoglobin's beta chain to another hydrophilic residue (lysine). Note: Compared to the sickle cell mutation, the clinical effects are not as significant since the change is from one hydrophilic to another hydrophilic residue versus the change in sickle cell anemia which involves a hydrophilic residue being replaced by a hydrophobic residue.
Hemoglobin E disease	A hemoglobinopathy that results from a mutation that leads to substitution of glutamic acid to lysine (hydrophilic to hydrophilic). Note: Compared to the sickle cell mutation, the clinical effects are not as significant since the change is from one hydrophilic to another hydrophilic residue versus the change in sickle cell anemia which involves a hydrophilic residue being replaced by a hydrophobic residue.
Hemoglobin H	An abnormal hemoglobin (beta chain tetramer) that is the result of excess B-chain production due to marked underproduction of alpha chains in severe alpha thalassemia.
Hemoglobin S disease	A hemoglobinopathy. Homozygous (Hb-SS) is sickle cell disease (symptomatic) and heterozygous is Sickle cell trait (usually asymptomatic). Hemoglobin S is the result of a mutation that changes the glutamic acid (hydrophilic) residue on the beta chain into valine (hydrophobic residue). The hydrophobic residue repels surrounding water and ultimately induces the deoxy hemoglobin molecules to polymerize, deforming the the red blood cell (sickle shaped).
Hemoglobinopathy	Genetic diseases that are associated with abnormal hemoglobins due to a mutation that usually leads to a structural abnormality in the hemoglobin molecule. Examples include sickle cell disease (HbSS), HbSC, HbE, and HbCC disease. In contrast to hemoglobinopathies, the defect in thalassemias leads to underproduction of the globin chains rather than a structural abnormality.

Hemolytic anemia	A subtype of anemia that is due to RBC hemolysis. 2 main types: Intravascular (can see schistocytes in PB) & Extravascular (can see spherocytes in PB). Lab findings include a low Hb and Hct, elevated reticulocyte count, increased bilirubin (mainly indirect bilirubin), hemoglobinemia, hemoglobinuria and sometimes hemosiderinuria. Decreased haptoglobin can also be seen and is more prominent in intravascular hemolysis. Causes may be congenital or inherited (e.g. sickle cell disease, hereditary spherocytosis, pyruvate kinase deficiency and G6PD deficiency) or acquired (infection-associated, immune-associated (Coombs positive), hypersplenism-associated, burn injury associated, or mechanical valve associated. Certain aspects of intravascular hemolysis such as schistocytes could also be seen in Microangiopathic Hemolytic Anemias which include DIC, TTP, and HUS.
Hemolytic uremic syndrome	Also known as HUS, it is a microangiopathic hemolytic anemia that is characterized by Renal failure (uremia) and thrombocytopenia. Mostly seen in children and preceded by diarrhea caused by E. coli O157:H7. Similar to TTP remember the mneumonic "Brain FART" which is Brain for neurologic problems (more commonly associated with TTP than HUS), F for Fever, A for Anemia, R for Renal failure (more commonly associated with HUS than TTP), and T for Thrombocytopenia.
Hemolytic disease of the newborn	Also known as HDN, it is an alloimmune reaction of maternal IgG molecules (directed against fetal RBC antigens) that cross the placenta and induce hemolysis and destrcution of the fetal RBCs.
Hemophilia	A group of hereditary genetic coagulation disorders that includes Hemophilia A, Hemophilia B, and Hemophilia C. Hemophilia A and B are X-linked disorders while Hemophilia C is an autosomal disorder. Hemophilia A is the most common form of the disorder and is characterized by Factor VIII deficiency. Hemophilia B is less common and is characterized by Factor IX deficiency. Hemophilia C is a lack of Factor XI. Symptoms may vary in severity but usually consist of internal and/or external bleeding (e.g. large joint bleeds).
Hemophilia A	An inherited X-linked bleeding disorder resulting from Factor VIII deficiency. It is the most common form of hemophilia. Symptoms vary depending on the severity and can include hemarthrosis, hematuria, epistaxis, bruising, and prolonged bleeding from cuts or tooth extraction. Typically the patient will have an elevated PTT and normal PT and bleeding time. Serum level of Factor VIII is also decreased. Treatment includes replacement of Factor VIII.
Hemophilia B	An inherited X-linked bleeding disorder resulting from Factor IX deficiency. Less common than Hemophilia A. Symptoms are similar to Hemophilia A (see Hemophilia A). The patient will have an elevated PTT and normal PT and bleeding time. Confirmed by low serum levels of Factory IX. Hemophilia B is treated with replacement of Factor IX.
Hemophilia C	A mild form of hemophilia that has an autosomal inheritance pattern characterized by Factor XI deficiency. Symptoms can be similar to Hemophilia A and B with the exception of hemarthrosis, which is a distinguishing feature. The disease is almost exclusively in Jews of Ashkenazi decent. Because the disease is mild, typically no treatment is required. Some cases such as pre-surgical patients, have been treated with FFP or recombinant Factor XI as necessary.
Hemosiderin	A form of iron-complexed to ferritin or other substances. This form of iron is not present in the blood and can be seen in tissue deposits and other sites. Hemosiderin is a major form of iron storage in the marrow and liver. Hemosiderin can increase abnormally in tissues or body fluids after hemorrhage. Hemosiderin is confirmed by stains for iron such as Prussian blue.
Heparin	Also known as unfractionated heparin, it is a widely used anticoagulant that is also naturally occurring in mast cells and basophils. Effective at preventing the formation of blood clots and is generally used for acute coronary syndrome, atrial fibrillation, deep-vein thrombosis, and etc. Heparin and its low molecular weight derivatives binds to the enzyme antithrombin (AT) that results in its activation which leads to the inactivation of thrombin and other proteases involved in blood clotting, most notably factor Xa. It is monitored by checking the PTT. A very notable and severe complication of unfractionated heparin is heparin-induced thrombocytopenia (HIT).
Hepcidin	A protein that is produced by the liver and acts as a major regulator of iron homeostasis. Hepcidin inhibits iron absorption from the small intestine and inhibits the release of iron from macrophages by binding the iron channel Ferroportin. Hence, when iron stores are low (such as Iron deficiency anemia) Hepcidin levels will decrease enabling iron absoprtion. In contrast, Hepcidin levels will increase in conditions that are not linked to low iron stores (e.g. Anemia of Chronic disease).
Hereditary elliptocytosis	A congenital RBC structural membrane disorder that is usually Autosomal Dominant and leads to increased numbers of RBCs with an elliptical shape (oval shaped). The defect is usually associated with a cytoskeletal scaffold of the RBC membrane. Mutations in the Spectrin genes (Spectrin protein is a structural protein) is the most common finding. Severe cases can lead to a hemolytic anemia.

Hereditary spherocytosis	A congenital RBC structural membrane disorder that is usually Autosomal Dominant and leads to increased numbers of RBCs with spherical shape (round with no central pallor). The defect is usually associated with a cytoskeletal scaffold of the RBC membrane. Mutations in the Spectrin genes (Spectrin protein is a strcutural protein), Ankyrin gene, Band 3 or Band 4.2 are the most common findings. Severe cases can lead to a hemolytic anemia. Usually there is an increase in MCHC. Additionally, the cells are more fragile and will give a positive osmotic fragility test result.
Hirudin	Belongs to the class of bivalent direct thrombin inhibitors, which also include Bivalirudin, Lepirudin, and Desirudin. Called bivalent because they bind both the active site and an allosteric site on the thrombin molecule to prevent coagulation. Mainly used to treat Heparin-Induced Thrombocytopenia. The drug is cleared by the kidney.
Histiocytes	This usually refers to tissue macrophages (monocytes that have left the blood and entered tissue). Histiocytes are antigen presenting cells that have phagocytic capabilities. 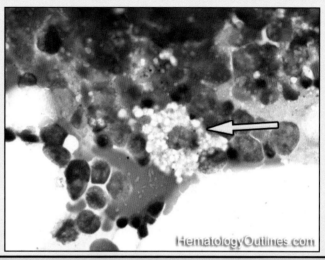
Hodgkin lymphoma	An indolent B-cell lymphoma that usually presents in supradiaphragmatic areas (above the diaphragm such as supraclavicular lymph nodes or anterior mediastinum). There is a bimodal age distribution (most patients present in their 20s and 50s). Four main subtypes are: Nodular Sclerosis, Mixed Cellularity, Lymphocyte-rich, and Lymphocyte-depleted. The hallmark of all classical Hodgkin lymphomas is the Reed-Sternberg cell (RS cell) which usually have the following immunophenotype: dim PAX5+, CD30+, CD15+, CD20-, OCT2- and BOB1-. 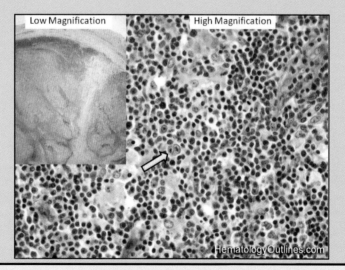
Homocysteine	This is the metabolite of the amino acid methionine. Homocysteine may be converted back to methionine with tetrahydrofolate (THF) as a cofactor, and THF is generated with the aid of vitamin B12. Hence, Hyperhomocyteinemia can be a result of vitamin B12 and/or folate deficiency, and has been linked to cardiovascular diseases. See vitamin B12 and Folate deficiency.

Howell-Jolly bodies	These are basophilic nuclear remnants (fragments of chromatin/DNA) in RBCs. Mostly seen in post-splenectomy patients or those with asplenia. Commonly seen in adults with Sickle Cell disease (Hb SS) since these patients have undergone autosplenectomy by the time they reach their adulthood. Remember as opposed to "HEinz" bodies which start with "HE" and stands for HEmoglobin, Howell-Jolly Bodies don't start with "HE" and are rather DNA or nuclear remnants. 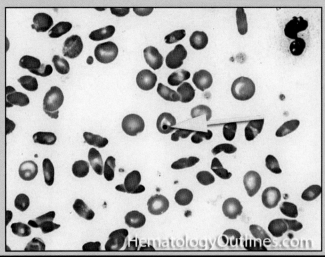
HUS	Also known as hemolytic uremic syndrome, it is a microangiopathic hemolytic anemia that is characterized by renal failure (uremia) and thrombocytopenia. Mostly seen in children and preceded by diarrhea caused by E. coli O157:H7. Similar to TTP remember the mneumonic "Brain FART" which is Brain for neurologic problems (more commonly associated with TTP than HUS), F for Fever, A for Anemia, R for Renal failure (more commonly associated with HUS than TTP), and T for Thrombocytopenia.
Hypersegmented neutrophils	These are neutrophils with more than 5 lobes (so 6 or more lobes. Recall, normal neutrophils should have 3-5 lobes). Hypersegmented neutrophils are most commonly associated with B12 or Folate deficiency (two common causes of a macrocytic anemia). 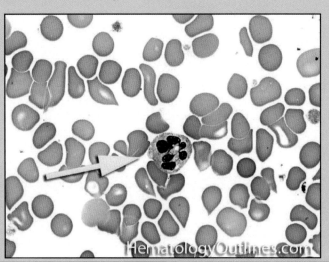

Hypogranular	This usually refers to neutrophils and platelets with decreased number of granules. Increased numbers of hypogranular neutrophils (dysplastic neutrophil) may be indicative of an underlying myelodysplastic syndrome.
IFE	Also known as immunofixation electrophoresis, it is an antibody-based method to detect and characterize clonal M-spikes noted on SPEP in patients with suspected plasma cell or B-cell neoplasms. This method reveals the M-spike as clonal with IgG, IgA, or IgM (rarely IgE or IgD) molecules that are either kappa or lambda light chain-restricted. (also known as a clonal antibody from a clonal neoplastic process such as a plasma cell neoplasm or a B-cell lymphoma). Note: IgG and IgA clones are typically associated with a plasma cell neoplasm (e.g. plasma cell myeloma or MGUS, etc.) while IgM clones may be related to Waldenstrom Macroglobulinemia which is typically associated with lymphoplasmacytic lymphoma.
Imatinib	Also known as Gleevec, it is a tyrosine kinase inhibitor used in treatment of CML by inhibiting the Philadelphia chromosome's tyrosine kinase product (ABL1).
Immunoblasts	Immunoblasts can be of B-cell or T-cell origin and reside in the perifollicular zones of secondary lymphoid tissue (such as lymph node) where they are morphologically indistinguishable. They are large cells with abundant cytoplasm, large nucleus with open chromatin, and a single centralized large nucleolus. They are part of the developmental stage of lymphocytes which follow the presentation of an antigen by MHC class II positive antigen presenting cells.
Immunoglobulin	The term is sometimes interchangeably used with antibody, a protein that is produced by B-cells (in terminally differentiated B-cells known as plasma cells these immunoglobulins are produced and secreted and are not cell surface bound) which recognize and bind to other proteins or substances (foreign or self antigens). Antibodies can be part of an immune response and help eradicate viruses and bacteria or may be part of an autoimmune destructive processes in hematology such as autoimmune hemolytic anemia or immune mediated platelet destruction (e.g. ITP). The different classes of antibodies are usually based on their heavy chains (e.g. IgA, IgG, IgE, IgD, and IgM).
Infectious mononucleosis	A disease that is usually due to Epstein Barr Virus (EBV). More common in younger patients and may present with lymphadenopathy and in severe cases with organomegaly (hepatomegaly and/or splenomegaly). The lymphadenopathy may sometimes mimic a lymphoma.
INR	Also known as International Normalized Ratio, it is a method to standardize the PT due to the variations between different batches of manufacturer's tissue factor that are used in the PT test. The normal range for INR is 0.8-1.2. Risk of bleeding increases with elevated INRs (see PT. see Coumadin.)
International Normalized Ratio	Also known as INR, it is a method to standardize the PT due to the variations between different batches of manufacturer's tissue factor that are used in the PT test. The normal range for INR is 0.8-1.2. Risk of bleeding increases with elevated INRs (see PT and coumadin).

Iron deficiency anemia	A microcytic anemia (MCV < 80)
JAK2	Also known as Janus Kinase 2, it is a protein whose signaling is involved in many receptor families including but not limited to erythropoietin and thrombopoietin receptors. Mutation of JAK2 has been identified in many myeloproliferative neoplasms such as polycythemia vera, essential thrombocythemia and primary myelofibrosis.
Kell	An RBC antigen group that contains immunogenic RBC antigens which may cause transfusion reactions or hemolytic disease of the newborn (HDN).
LA	Also known as Lupus anticoagulant, it is an immunoglobulin that binds to phospholipids and interferes with the coagulation process in vitro leading to a prolonged PTT. Although the PTT is elevated in LA, the name is a misnomer because it is not an anticoagulant but rather causing thrombosis in vivo. Also most patients with LA do not have Lupus (SLE) . When presented with a prolonged PTT, a mixing study is performed. If the PTT is corrected, then LA is excluded. However, if the clotting time is still prolonged, then the presence of an inhibitor is confirmed, which includes LA. Confirmation of LA is then confirmed through a phospholipid sensitive test such as Dilute Russell's Viper Venom Time (see dRVVT).
Large cell lymphoma	Includes diffuse large b-cell lymphoma (DLBCL) and anaplastic large cell lymphoma (usually a T-cell lymphoma). By definition, the neoplastic cells in these lymphomas are typically three times the size or larger than small mature lymphocytes.

Large granular lymphocytes	Also known as LGLs, these are T-lymphocytes with an increased amount of cytoplasm and multiple small red cytoplasmic granules. Increased numbers could be seen in reactive conditions (such as infections) or an indolent neoplastic process such as the T-cell leukemia known as T-LGL leukemia.
Left shifted	Usually refers to seeing less mature cells of a certain lineage. Commonly refers to seeing an increased amount of less mature myeloid (granulocytic) precursors such as myelocytes, metamyelocytes and bands in the blood or bone marrow.
Lenalidomide	Brand name: Revlimid. It is a chemotherapy drug used to treat plasma cell myeloma and myelodysplastic syndromes (MDS), specifically in patients with deletion 5q with or without additional cytogenetic abnormalities. Side effects include marrow toxicity resulting in neutropenia and thrombocytopenia.
Leukemia	Literally means white blood and refers to a neopastic hematopoietic neoplasm of lymphoid or myeloid origin that involves the peripheral blood. They can be immature (Acute) or mature/maturing (Chronic). Acute leukemias include Acute Myeloid Leukemia (AML) and Acute Lymphoid Leukemia (ALL). Examples of maturing/mature leukemias include Chronic Myelogenous Leukemia (CML) and Chronic Lymphocytic Leukemia (CLL).
Leukocytes	Means "White cells" and refers to the White Blood Cells (WBCs) which include Granulocytes (Neutrophil, Eosinophil, Basophil), monocytes, and lymphocytes and their precursors. The leukocyte precursors (e.g. promyelocyte, myelocyte, metamyelocyte) are usually seen in the bone marrow and absent in blood of normal individuals.
Leukoerythroblastosis	Refers to the presence of white blood cell precursors and nucleated RBCs in the peripheral blood. This may be due to an underlying marrow infiltrative process, severe infection or severe hemolysis.

Lipocyte	These are fat cells that are typically seen as empty spaces in the bone marrow. The amount of non-fat (cellular) portion of the marrow is the marrow's estimated cellularity. Normal cellularity in people between the age of 15 to 75 is expected to be 100 minus the patient's age (in percentage). Hence, 70% marrow cellularity in a 30 year old patient is the expected norm (100-30=70%). While 70% cellularity in a 75 year old patient is considered a hypercellular marrow.
Liver disease coagulopathy	Coagulopathy due to liver disease. Most coagulation factors are made in the liver (majority are made in the liver hepatocytes while factor VIII is made in the reticuloendothelial cells in liver or other sites). Hence, in end-stage liver disease (e.g. cirrhosis) deficiency of these factors usually leads to coagulopathy.
Low molecular weight heparin	Low molecular weight derivative of unfractionated heparin (e.g. enoxaparin, dalteparin, tinzaparin) that prevents coagulation by targeting factor Xa activity rather than antithrombin activity, as in unfractionated heparin. Usually does not require monitoring with PTT (as opposed to unfractionated heparin) and markedly reduces the risk of Heparin-Induced Thrombocytopenia (HIT). Can be monitored with anti-factor Xa assay in certain clinical scenarios.
Lupus anticoagulant	Also known as LA, it is an immunoglobulin that binds to phospholipids and interferes with the coagulation process in vitro leading to a prolonged PTT. Although the PTT is elevated in LA, the name is a misnomer because it is not an anticoagulant but rather causing thrombosis in vivo. Also most patients with LA do not have Lupus (SLE) . When presented with a prolonged PTT, a mixing study is performed. If the PTT is corrected, then LA is excluded. However, if the clotting time is still prolonged, then the presence of an inhibitor is confirmed, which includes LA. Confirmation of LA is then confirmed through a phospholipid sensitive test such as Dilute Russell's Viper Venom Time (see dRVVT).
Lymph node	A peripheral or secondary lymphoid tissue where B-cell migrate to complete their maturation (B-cells undergo somatic hypermutation and class switching of heavy chains in the germinal center of secondary follicles in lymph nodes and other secondary lymphoid tissues such as Mucosa-Associated Lymphoid Tissue and spleen). Mature B-cells could ultimately become plasma cells or memory B-cells in the lymph nodes or other secondary lymphoid tissues. Additionally, the interfollicular areas of these secondary lymphoid tissues are mostly comprised of mature T-cells.
Lymphoblast	Immature cell of the lymphoid lineage. In an abnormal neoplastic disorder such as acute lymphoblastic leukemia/lymphoma (ALL) they are either of a B-cell (B-ALL) or T-cell (T-cell) origin.

Lymphocytes	A type of leukocyte or WBC (second most prevalent WBC in a normal peripheral blood. Most prevalent is neutrophils followed by lymphocytes followed by monocytes, followed by eosinophils and ultimately basophils which are rarely seen). The three main types of lymphocytes include B-cells, T-cells and NK-cells. 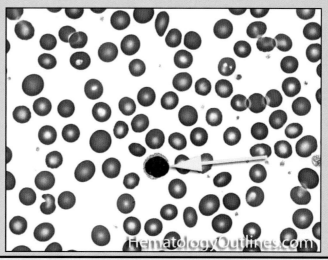
Lymphocytosis	This typically refers to an increase in the absolute count of lymphocytes in the peripheral blood. This is also sometimes referred to as "absolute lymphocytosis" where the absolute count is usually greater than 4000 x 10^3/μL. Common causes of lymphocytosis are infections (usually viral but sometimes bacterial such as B. pertussis) and B cell neoplasms especially CLL. 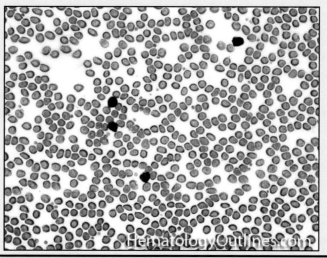
Lymphoma	A neoplastic malignancy of lymphoid origin (B-cell, T-cell or NK cell in origin) that involves some tissue (e.g. lymph node, spleen, liver, stomach, etc.). The T-cell and NK cell lymphomas are typically Non-Hodgkin lymphomas while B-cell lymphomas can be either Non-Hodgkin or Hodgkin lymphomas.

Lymphoma mnemonic	A mnemonic for common translocations associated with several mature B-cell lymphomas. 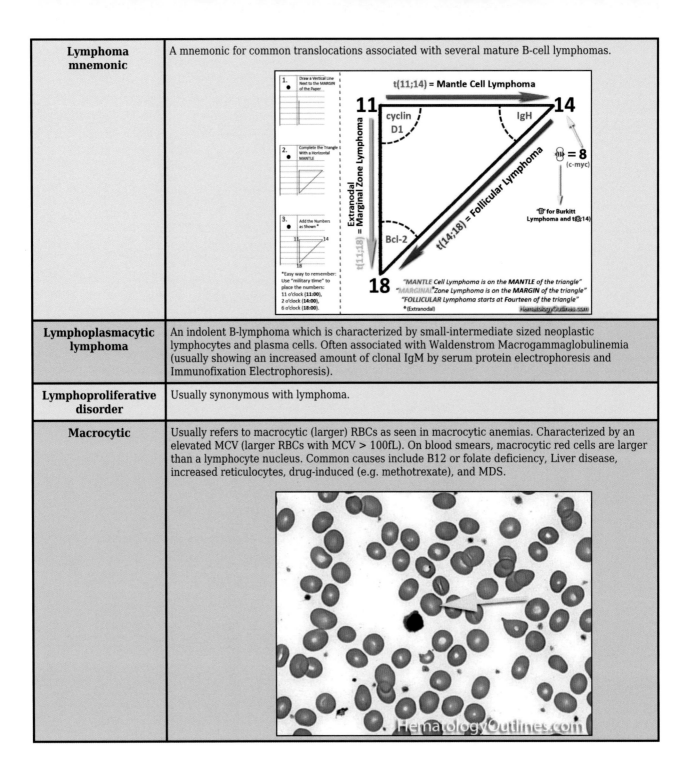
Lymphoplasmacytic lymphoma	An indolent B-lymphoma which is characterized by small-intermediate sized neoplastic lymphocytes and plasma cells. Often associated with Waldenstrom Macrogammaglobulinemia (usually showing an increased amount of clonal IgM by serum protein electrophoresis and Immunofixation Electrophoresis).
Lymphoproliferative disorder	Usually synonymous with lymphoma.
Macrocytic	Usually refers to macrocytic (larger) RBCs as seen in macrocytic anemias. Characterized by an elevated MCV (larger RBCs with MCV > 100fL). On blood smears, macrocytic red cells are larger than a lymphocyte nucleus. Common causes include B12 or folate deficiency, Liver disease, increased reticulocytes, drug-induced (e.g. methotrexate), and MDS.

Macrophages	Monocytes that have left the blood and entered tissue to serve various functions including phagocytosis of debris and modulate the immune response. HematologyOutlines.com
Mantle cell lymphoma	An intermediately (between a low grade and high grade lymphoma) aggressive CD5 positive CD23 negative B-cell lymphoma that is usually due to t(11;14) leading to the overexpression of Cyclin D1 (BCL1). This is in contrast to CLL which is usually CD5+, CD23+ and BCL1 (Cyclin D1) negative. Low Magnification High Magnification CD20+ CD5+ HematologyOutlines.com

Mast cells	They have many similarities to basophils. Masts cells are usually noted in tissue and bone marrow but absent from peripheral blood (unlike basophils which are in bone marrow and peripheral blood). Mast cells can release substances such as histamine in allergic reactions. Neoplastic mast cells cause cutaneous and systemic mastocytosis. Both normal and abnormal mast cells are typically positive for Mast cell tryptase and CD117 (C-Kit). However, most abnormal mast cells may aberrantly express CD2 and CD25 (T-cell markers). 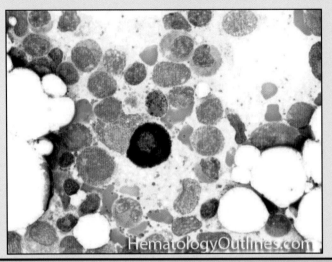
May-Hegglin anomaly	Due to Myosin Heavy Chain 9 (MYH-9) mutation. Patients usually show Döhle-like bodies in their neutrophils along with giant platelets in peripheral blood. 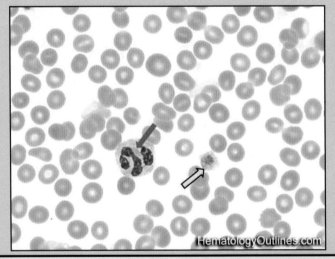
MDS	Stands for myelodysplastic syndrome. A heterogeneous group of chronic myeloid neoplasms which usually share the following features: cytopenia (decrease blood counts such as anemia, thrombocytopenia, or neutropenia) with the exception of MDS with isolated 5q- which may show an increase in platelets), lack of splenomegaly and a hypercellular marrow. The most common MDS include RAEB-I, RAEB-II, RCUD (e.g. RA or RARS), RCMD, and MDS with isolated 5q-. RAEB have the worst prognosis (higher liklihod of transforming into AML) while MDS with isolated 5q- has the best prognosis.
MDS with isolated 5q-	Also known as MDS with isolated 5q deletion, this is a type of MDS characteristically showing normal or elevated platelet count with a bone marrow displaying increased numbers of hypolobated megakaryocytic along with erythroid hypoplasia. The normal or increased platelet count is unusual amongst MDS, and when the 5q- is the sole cytogenetic abnormality, the prognosis is better than most MDS. These patients are usually treated with lenalidomide.

Megakaryoblast	Immature (blast) form of the megakaryocytic cell lineage (the lineage responsible for making platelets). Increased numbers may be seen in certain AMLs (M7: Acute Megakaryoblastic Leukemia) and AML look-a-likes such as Transient Myelopoiesis which are both more commonly seen in Down Syndrome patients. 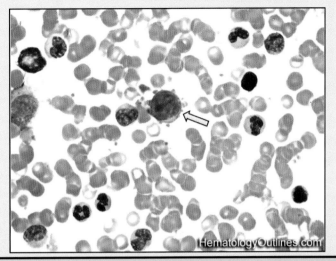
Megakaryocytes	Usually the largest cells in the bone marrow that are 10 to 15 times larger than a typical red blood cell. The maturing megakaryocyte grows in size and replicates its DNA without nuclear division resulting in a very large, lobulated, nucleus with many copies of the usual complement of DNA, as much as 64 times most cells. They are multinucleated and responsible for making platelets. 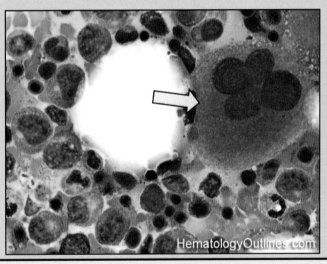
Megaloblastic anemia	A cause of macrocytic anemia characterized by large immature RBC precursors (megaloblastoid RBC precursors) in the bone marrow that is the result of impairment in DNA synthesis during RBC production. Common causes include Vitamin B12 deficiency, folate deficiency, chemotherapy-induced (e.g. Methotrexate, 6-Mercaptopurine or Cytosine Arabinoside), and certain malignancies (e.g. MDS).

Megaloblastoid erythroid changes	These are larger than usual erythroid (RBC) precursors with relatively immature nuclear features for the maturity of the cytoplasm (nuclear/cytoplasmic maturation asynchrony). Causes include certain vitamin deficiencies (e.g. B12 or Folate deficiency), drug effects such as methotrexate or due to an underlying myelodysplastic syndrome (MDS).
Metamyelocyte	A myeloid (granulocytic) precursor that follows the myelocyte stage and precedes the band stage in the maturation steps of granulocytes. There is indentation of the nucleus but less than 50% of its diameter (as opposed to a band which has an indentation of >50% of the nucleus diameter).
Metastasis	Distant spread of a malignancy (e.g. primary malignancy of lung spreading to the liver or bone, etc.). Note: benign neoplasms usually do not metastasize.
Methemoglobin	Also known as MetHb. The iron in the heme moiety of this hemoglobin molecule is in the Fe^{+++} state and cannot release the bound oxygen. Note: normal hemoglobin's heme moiety is Fe^{++} and able to release the bound oxygen.
Methylmalonic acid	Also known as MMA, it is a Dicarboxylic acid. When linked to coenzyme A, methylmalonyl-CoA is converted to succinyl-CoA using vitamin B12 as a cofactor in the Kreb cycle. Vitamin B12 deficiency causes elevated levels of methylmalonic acid (MMA). See vitamin B12 deficiency.
MGUS	Monoclonal Gammopathy of Uncertain Significance are part of plasma cell neoplasms and thought to be precursors to plasma cell myeloma. Similar to the other plasma cell neoplams, they typically display an M-spike on Serum Protein Electrophoresis and shown to be clonal by IFE.
Microangiopathic hemolytic anemia	As the name (microangio) implies, it is a small vessel disease associated hemolytic anemia (intravascular hemolytic anemias). Examples include HUS, TTP, DIC and sometimes due to malignant hypertension.

Microcytic	Usually refers to microcytic (small) RBCs that are seen in microcytic anemia. These are anemias with small RBCs (MCV of < 80).

Micromegakaryocytes	These are small abnormal (dysplastic) non-lobated megakaryocytes that are usually associated with an underlying Myeloid neoplasm such as myelodysplastic syndrome.

Microspherocyte	Small round RBCs with no central pallor that may be seen in in blood smears from patients with immune-mediated hemolytic anemia, burn injuries, and hereditary spherocytosis.
Mixing study (1:1 mix)	A laboratory test used to distinguish factor deficiencies versus factor inhibitors such as lupus anticoagulant. The test is performed by mixing the patient's plasma with a known normal control plasma in a 1:1 ratio. If the 1:1 mixing study results in the correction of PT and/or PTT, then the patient most likely has a factor deficiency. Follow-up factor assays can be performed to further identify the deficiency. No correction mostly likely indicates the presence of a factor inhibitor (most likely an antibody). For patients on anticoagulant therapy, the test should not be performed until the anticoagulant is discontinued. In some situations, the inhibitors are time-dependent, therefore, the 1:1 mix is incubated for 2 hours at 37° C first. An example of such a time-dependent inhibitor is the Factor VIII inhibitor.
MMA	Also known as Methylmalonic acid, it is a Dicarboxylic acid. When linked to coenzyme A, methylmalonyl-CoA is converted to succinyl-CoA using vitamin B12 as a cofactor in the Kreb cycle. Vitamin B12 deficiency causes elevated levels of methylmalonic acid (MMA). See vitamin B12 deficiency.

Monocytes	A type of white blood cell (derived from the myeloid lineage). These are usually the largest circulating cells in the blood and usually 2-3 times the size of a mature lymphocyte. Their nucleus is usually folded, and there is a large amount of light blue cytoplasm and commonly show cytoplasmic vacuoles. Monocytes that leave the blood and enter tissue are called macrophages.
Mott cells	These are enlarged plasma cells with multiple cytoplasmic globules which are comprised of immunoglobulins. Mott cells can be seen in certain non-neoplastic (e.g. certain autoimmune diseases) and neoplastic (e.g. plasma cell neoplasms such as plasma cell myeloma, also known as mutiple myeloma) processes.
MPN	A group of mature or maturing myeloid neoplasms that usually share the following features: Cytosis refers to the increase in various blood counts (red count, white count, platelet count) with the exception of Primary Myelofibrosis), splenomegaly (less common in ET patients), and hypercellular marrow (except in Primary Myelofibrosis or spent phase of the some MPNs). The most common MPNs include CML, PV, ET, and Primary Myelofibrosis. CML has the t(9;22) translocation (BCR/ABL1) while PV, ET and Primary Myelofibrosis usually show the JAK2 mutation.
Multiple myeloma	Also known as plasma cell myeloma. This is a plasma cell neoplasm that is usually characterized by increased numbers (10% or more) of monoclonal plasma cells in the bone marrow. Two main types: Asymptomatic (Smoldering) and Symptomatic (characterized by one or more of the following CRAB findings: Remember "CRAB", C for hyperCalcemia, R for Renal disease associated with multiple myeloma, A for Anemia associated with the multiple myeloma, and B for lytic Bone lesions).
Mycoses fungoides	Also known as MF, it is the most common skin lymphoproliferative disorder. These are usually CD4+ T-cell lymphomas with characteristic epidermotropism (neoplastic cells crawling up into the epidermis) and Pautrier's micro abscesses (collection of neoplastic cells around a dendritic cell in the epidermis).

Myeloblasts	An immatute (blast) form of the myeloid lineage. Normal bone marrow usually has a range of 1-3% myeloblasts. Increased numbers are usually secondary to an underlying myeloid neoplasm such as MDS (RAEB when there is < 20% myelobasts).
Myelocyte	A granulocytic precursor that follows promyelocyte in the maturation step of granulocytes. Recall maturation steps of granulocytes: myeloblast to promyelocyte to myelocyte to metamyelocyte to band and finally to segmented granulocyte.
Myelodysplastic syndrome	Also known as MDS, it is a heterogeneous group of chronic myeloid neoplasms which usually share the following features: cytopenia (decrease in number of a cell line in blood with the exception of MDS with isolated 5q- which may show an increase in platelets), lack of splenomegaly and a hypercellular marrow. The most common MDS include RAEB-I, RAEB-II, RCUD (e.g. RA or RARS), RCMD, and MDS with isolated 5q-. RAEB have the worst prognosis (higher liklihod of transforming into AML) while MDS with isolated 5q- has the best prognosis.
Myeloproliferative neoplasms	A group of mature or maturing myeloid neoplasms that usually share the following features: Cytosis (increase in a cell line in blood with the exception of primary myelofibrosis), splenomagly (less common in ET patients), and hypercellular marrow (except in primary myelofibrosis or spent phase of the some MPNs). The most common MPNs include CML, PV, ET, and primary myelofibrosis. CML has the t(9;22) translocation (BCR/ABL1) while PV, ET and primary myelofibrosis many show the JAK2 mutation.
Natural killer cell	Abbreviated as NK-cell. A cytotoxic lymphoid cell that is part of the innate immune system. Its cytotoxicity is due to its ability of releasing small cytotoxic granules such as perforin and granzymes. They have some similarities to the Cytotoxic CD8+ T-cells. However, unlike the T-cells, NK-cells do not express T-cell Receptors (TCRs), surface CD3 or CD5. They usually express CD56, CD16 and contain some relatively NK specific receptors such as CD94 and KIR (Killer-cell Immunoglobulin-like Receptor).

Necrosis	A type of cell death. As opposed to apoptosis which can be normal or abnormal, necrotic cell death is almost always abnormal. Common types of necrosis include coagulative necrosis (e.g. tumor necrosis), liquefactive necrosis (e.g. in brain post injury), caseous necrosis (grossly looks cheese-like and may be due to underling tuberculosis or fungal infection), fat necrosis, and hyaline vascular necrosis
Neoplasm	Usually refers to a clonal growth (tumor). These may be benign or malignant. Benign tumors include adenomas while malignant ones include carcinoma (epithelial), sarcoma (mesenchymal), melanoma (melanocytic), lymohoma and leukemia (hematopoietic).
Neutrophils	Also known as PMN (for polymorphonuclear), it belongs to the myeloid (granulocytic) cell lineage. Neutrophils usually increase in blood secondary to infection (esp. bacterial). As opposed to eosinophils and basophils, the granules in neutrophils are neutral (light pink) in color.
Non-Hodgkin lymphoma	These are mature/maturing neoplastic lymphoid cells (lymphoma) of either B-cell, NK-cell or T-cell lineage. Examples include Diffuse Large B-Cell Lymphoma (DLBCL) and follicular lymphoma which are of B-cell origin while Anaplastic Large Cell Lymhphoma (ALCL) and Peripheral T-Cell Lymphoma Not Otherwise Specified (PTCL-NOS) are of T-cell origin.
Normoblast	An erythroid precursor (nucleated form of erythroid).

Normochromic/normocytic erythrocytes	These are normal appearing mature RBCs and can be seen in normal individuals or those with certain anemias. As opposed to the immature erythroid precursors which are nucleated, the mature RBCs lack a nucleus and have a central pallor that is usually 1/3 of its diameter. The main function of the RBC is to carry oxygen through its hemoglobin molecules.
Normocytic	This refers to "normal size" mature RBCs or anemias with normocytic appearance (MCV 80-100 which is the normal range). These anemias include but are not limited to Hemolytic anemia, Sickle cell anemia, and Anemia of Chronic disease.
Nucleated red blood cells	These are also known as NRBC which are red blood cells who as the name implies have a nucleus (as opposed to normal mature RBCs that do not have a nucleus). Increased numbers of these less mature erythroid cells can be associated with an underlying infiltrative marrow process, leukoerythroblastic process and sometimes as a response to severe hemolysis.

Osteoblasts	Resident cells in the bone that are responsible for bone formation. May sometimes resemble plasma cells (which have a perinuclear cytoplasmic clearing, as opposed to the cytoplasmic clearing in osteoblasts that is away from the nucleus and more in the center of the cytoplasm).
Osteoclasts	Multinucleated resident cells in the bone that are responsible for bone resorption. May sometimes resemble other multinucleated cells in the bone marrow such as megakaryocytes (the nuclei of megakaryocytes are connected to each other while the nuclei of osteoclasts appear round and disconnected from one another).
Ovalocytes	Also sometimes referred to as elliptocytes are RBCs with an elongated or oval shape and may be secondary to hereditary elliptocytosis or iron deficiency anemia to name a few.

Pappenheimer bodies	Dense, blue-purple granules of iron found in the periphery of the cytoplasm of an RBC. Most commonly, they are associated with splenectomy, either surgical or as a complication of sickle cell anemia. They also can be seen in smears from patients with sideroblastic anemia, and hemolytic anemias. In contrast to Howell-Jolly (HJ) bodies that are a single, very round red cell inclusions, Pappenheimer bodies are smaller, more irregular in outline, and often are multiple per red blood cell. 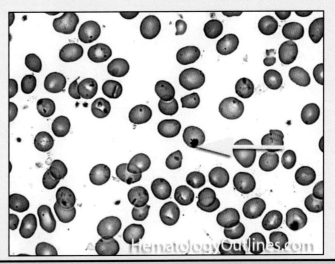
Paroxysmal cold hemoglobinuria	This a rare autoimmune hemolytic anemia that is due to cold reacting IgG antibodies to the RBC P antigen. These antibodies bind RBCs at cold temperature and with elevated temperature the bound red cells undergo a complement induced destruction (hemolysis). These biphasic unusual cold reacting IgGs are also known as Donath-Landsteiner antibodies. These patients may undergo hemolysis when exposed to cold temperature and present with hemoglobinuria. Peripheral blood may show some neutrophils with erythrophagocytosis. 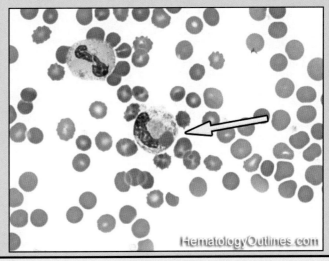
Paroxysmal Nocturnal hemoglobinuria	Also known as PNH, it is an acquired complement-induced hemolytic anemia that is due to a mutation of phosphatidylinositol glycan A (PIGA) gene (on chromosone X) which is resposible for making the cell membrane protein anchoring molecule glycosylphosphatidylinositol (GPI). Notably the gene is on chromosome X but unlike X-linked germline mutations (e.g. Hemophilia A) which almost exclusively involve males, this acquired mutation involves males and females equally. The diagnosis is made by flow cytometry and showing loss of CD55 (Complement decay accelerating factor) and CD59 (protectin which usually inhibits the complement membrane attack complex) on multiple blood cell types (RBCs and WBCs). These patients are also at an increased risk of thrombosis.

Pelger-Huet anomaly	A rare inherited condition due to lamin B receptor mutation in which most of the peripheral blood neutrophils present with bilobed nuclei connected with a thin filament of chromatin (similar to the bilobed nuclei noted on normal mature eosinophils but without the eosinophilic granules). In heterozygous individuals these neutrophils appear to maintain their function, and most of these individuals are asymptomatic (hence the term anomaly rather than disease). 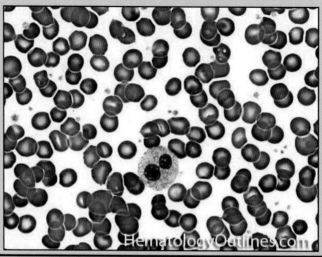
Plasma cell	This is a terminally differentiated B-cell that produces and secretes immunoglobulins (antibodies). Some B-cells in the peripheral lymphoid tissues (e.g. lymph node) further differentiate and become plasma cells. Normally plasma cells are not present in the peripheral blood and reside in secondary lymphoid tissues and other tissues such as the bone marrow. It has an eccentric nucleus with a "clock-face" chromatin pattern and abundant blue cytoplasm and a perinuclear clearing. 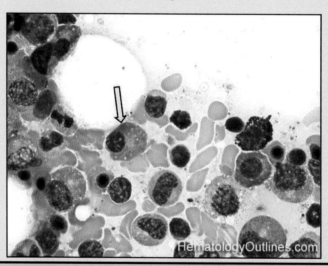
Plasma cell leukemia	This is a very aggressive plasma cell neoplasm with an increased number circulating plasma cells in the peripheral blood (usually >20% of WBCs).

Plasma cell myeloma	Also known as multiple myeloma, it is a plasma cell neoplasm that is usually characterized by increased numbers (10% or more) of monoclonal plasma cells in the bone marrow. Two main types: Asymptomatic (Smoldering) and Symptomatic (characterized by one or more of the following CRAB findings: Remember "CRAB", C for hyperCalcemia, R for Renal disease associated with multiple myeloma, A for Anemia associated with the multiple myeloma, and B for lytic Bone lesions).
Plasmacytoma	A plasma cell neoplasm that consists almost entirely of neoplastic plasma cells involving tissue outside of the bone marrow.
Plasminogen	Plasminogen is a zymogen produced by the liver and released into the circulation. Plasminogen is cleaved by enzymes such as tissue-plasminogen activator (t-PA) to form plasmin. Plasmin (a serine protease) is then responsible for degradation of fibrin clot, a process known as fibrinolysis.
Platelet granules	Platelet granules are present within platelets and released during platelet activation. There are three types of granules present within platelets: Alpha granules, Delta (dense) granules and Lysosomes. Alpha granules contain the larger molecules such as Platelet Factor 4 (PF4), Platelet-derived growth factor (PDGF), fibrinogen and some other clotting factors. The Delta (Dense) Granules contain the smaller molecules such as Serotonin, ADP, & Calcium. Mnemonic is Alpha stands for the "Bigger" molecules such as proteins and peptides, while Delta or Dense stands for "Diminutive" (tiny) molecules.
Platelets	Cellular fragments (2-3 μm in diameter which correlates to about 1/3 to 1/2 the size of a RBC) released from megakaryocytes into the blood and involved in hemostasis.
Pleuripotential hematopoietic stem cells	These stem cells are derived from totipotent stem cells and can differentiate into any of the hematopoetic cell lines (myeloid or lymphoid).

PNH	Paroxysmal nocturnal hemoglobinuria is an acquired complement-induced hemolytic anemia that is due to a mutation of phosphatidylinositol glycan A (PIGA) gene (on chromosone X) which is resposible for making the cell membrane protein anchoring molecule glycosylphosphatidylinositol (GPI). Notably the gene is on chromosome X but unlike X-linked germline mutations (e.g. Hemophilia A) which almost exclusively involve males, this acquired mutation involves males and females equally. The diagnosis is made by flow cytometry and showing loss of CD55 (Complement decay accelerating factor) and CD59 (protectin which usually inhibits the complement membrane attack complex) on multiple blood cell types (RBCs and WBCs). These patients are also at an increased risk of thrombosis.
Poikilocytosis	The presence in the blood of erythrocytes showing abnormal variation in "shape". Mnemonic is when compared to Anisocytosis. Both the words "Shape" and "Poikilocytosis" contain a "P". Therefore Poikilocytosis has to do with RBC Shape variation while Anisocytosis (No "P" in the word) has to do with variation of "size" (No "P" in the word). 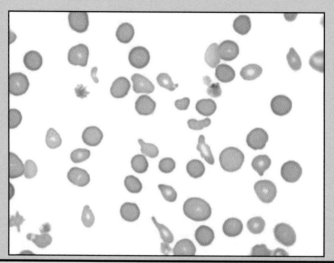
Polychromatophilic	Usually refers to the polychromatophilic RBC which is a less mature non-nucleated red blood cell with a light basophilic (light blue-purple) color on peripheral smear which is due to the presence of cytoplasmic RNA. Increased numbers may be seen in certain anemias such as hemolytic anemia in which earlier RBCs are being released by the reactive bone marrow in response to the anemia with the earlier release of these less mature RBCs into circulation. A special stain can highlight the RNA molecules in these cells and on the special stain these cell are known as reticulocytes. 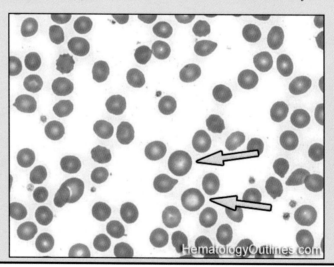

Polycythemia vera	A myeloprolifeartive neoplasm that usually carries the JAK2 mutation. Patients with this neoplasm typically present with splenomegaly, and some "cytosis" which is usually in the form of an elevated hematrocrit/hemoglobin with low EPO levels. The bone marrow is usually hypercellular similar to many of the other myeloproliferative neoplasms.
Proerythroblast	The earliest erythrocyte precursor in the erythrocyte series which usually contains a large nucleus with several nucleoli and high nucleus/cytoplasm ratio (meaning very little cytoplasm).
Promyelocytes	A granulocytic precursor that follows the myeloblast stage and precedes the myelocyte stage. They usually contain one or more nuceloli and a few or many coarse, reddish-purple, azurophilic (primary) granules.
Protein C	Protein C is an inactive enzyme form (zymogen) of activated protein C (APC) which plays an important role in anticoagulation. Protein C is a vitamin K dependent protein produced by the liver. Protein C is activated by thrombin, with Protein S as a cofactor, to from APC, a serine protease. APC then acts to inhibit the activation of Factor V and VIII. Protein C deficiency ranges from mild to severe. Depending on the type of deficiency (heterozygous or homozygous), it can lead to an increased risk of thrombosis.
Protein S	Protein S is a vitamin K dependent glycoprotein produced in the endothelium. It is important in anticoagulation because it acts as a cofactor in the activation of Protein C (see Protein C). Protein S deficiency, caused by a mutation in the PROS1 gene, is rare but can lead to an increased risk of thrombosis.

Prothrombin time	Also known as PT, it is a laboratory test used to measure the integrity of the extrinsic coagulation pathway and commonly used to monitor warfarin (Coumadin) therapy. Normal range: 10-13 seconds. It is sensitive to detecting deficiencies in the extrinsic pathway such as factor VII and common pathway factors I, II, V, and X. Note: Common pathway coagulation factors effect both PT and PTT). The test is performed by taking citrated plasma to clot at 37° C after the addition of calcium. Tissue factor is then added and the time it takes to clot is measured. The resultant PT is normalized with the International Normalized Ratio (INR) (see INR). PT is typically increased in Coumadin therapy, vitamin K deficiency, liver disease, DIC, and deficiencies in extrinsic or common pathway coagulation factor(s).
Pseudo-Gaucher cells	Pseudo-Gaucher cells are histiocytes with cytoplasmic needle-like inclusions, resembling histiocytes noted in Gaucher disease (Gaucher cells). These pseudo-Gaucher cells have been shown in a variety of diseases including but not limited to CML, multiple myeloma, and ALL.
Pseudothrombocytopenia	Pseudo-thrombocytopenia is an artifactual clumping of platelets that can occur after exposure to EDTA. The clumping occurs only in the test tube with EDTA and may be associated with an antibody that reacts to platelet antigens only in the presence of EDTA. Citrated blood can be used to get an accurate platelet count when EDTA causes this problem.
PT	Also known as prothrombin time, this is a laboratory test used to measure the integrity of the extrinsic coagulation pathway and commonly used to monitor warfarin (Coumadin) therapy. Normal range: 10-13 seconds. It is sensitive to detecting deficiencies in the extrinsic pathway such as factor VII and common pathway factors I, II, V, and X (Note: Common pathway coagulation factors effect both PT and PTT). The test is performed by taking citrated plasma to clot at 37° C after the addition of calcium. Tissue factor is then added and the time it takes to clot is measured. The resultant PT is normalized with the International Normalized Ratio (INR) (see INR). PT is typically increased in Coumadin therapy, vitamin K deficiency, liver disease, DIC, and deficiencies in extrinsic or common pathway coagulation factor(s).
PTT	Activated Partial Thromboplastin Time is a laboratory test that measures the integrity of the intrinsic pathway of coagulation and commonly used for monitoring heparin therapy. It is sensitive to detecting deficiencies in factors involved in the intrinsic pathway such as factor VIII, IX, and XI, common pathway such as factor X or phospholipid-dependent inhibitors such as lupus anticoagulants. As noted above, it is also prolonged if certain anticoagulants such as heparin are present. The test is performed by taking citrated plasma to clot at 37° C after the addition of calcium (a set amount of phospholipid is also added but no Tissue Factor is added so it will not evaluate the extrinsic pathway). PTT could also be used comparatively in mixing studies when one suspects factor deficiency or presence of inhibitors. In a patient with prolonged PTT (& normal PT), first the presence of heparin must be excluded. Once heparin is excluded, the patient's plasma can be mixed with a known normal plasma sample to see if the PTT corrects. Correction of the PTT in such setting is suggestive of a factor deficiency while lack of correction may imply presence of an inhibitor (antibody), such as lupus anticoagulant.
RBC	Also called red blood cell or erythrocyte, it is the most common type of blood cell in the body. Its role is to deliver oxygen via the hemoglobin molecule to various tissues and organs.

Reactive lymphocytes	Previously referred to as atypical lymphocytes. These large lymphocytes may be increased in the peripheral blood smear in certain inflammatory conditions such as an underlying viral infection (e.g. EBV induced mononucleosis, the lymphocytes look so large that they start resembling monocytes). They usually have increased amount of cytoplasm which wraps or hugs the surrounding RBCs. Reactive lymphocytes are typically CD8+ T-cells.
Red blood cell	Also called RBC or erythrocyte, these are the most common type of blood cell in the body. Its role is to deliver oxygen via the hemoglobin molecule to various tissues and organs.
Refractory anemia	A subtype of MDS under the category of Refractory Cytopenia with Unilineage Dysplasia.
Reticulin fibrosis	A type of fibrosis (reticulin usually refers to type III collagen) made evident by special reticulin stains. Marrows may show increased reticulin for various reasons including metastatic tumors, lymphoma, and clonal disorders of the marrow (MDS, AML, MPN). Extensive increases in reticulin are characteristic of primary myelofibrosis and a common complication of other MPN.

Reticulocytes	Reticulocytes are immature RBCs that do no contain nuclei but have increased amounts of RNA. On normal peripheral blood smears stained with Wright-Giemsa they appear as polychromatophilic cells (light purple/blue cells are the polychromatophilic cells versus the more mature RBCs stain pink/red) and with special stains (such as supravital stain) one could highlight the excess RNA within the cytoplasm of these RBCs known as reticulocytes. Normal range for reticulocytes in the peripheral blood is 0.5-1.5%. Increased reticulocytes can be seen in the setting of anemias that are due to desctruction of RBCs (such as in autoimmune hemolytic anemia) which causes the marrow to increase production of newer RBCs. Low recticulocytes are usually indicative of marrow underproduction and can be caused by chemotherapy, aplastic anemia, pernicious anemia, bone marrow malignancies, vitamin and mineral deficiencies, chronic diseases, or lack of erythropoietin production. 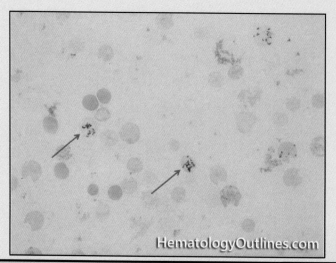
Reticuloendothelial cells	These cells are part of the immune system that comprises certain phagocytic cells such as monocytes and macrophages within the reticular connective tissue as noted in the spleen, liver and the lymph node.
Ring sideroblasts	Abnormal nucleated RBCs with granules of iron accumulated in perinuclear mitochondria, which can be seen by microscopy after special iron stains such as Prussian Blue. Increased ring sideroblasts are a diagnostic feature of certain disease states such as the Myelodysplastic syndrome Refractory Anemia with Ring Sideroblasts. Other causes of ring sideroblasts include copper deficiency, and zinc toxicity (which could induce copper deficiency). Ring sideroblasts are specifically defined as sideroblasts encircled by 5 or more iron granules and surrounding at least 1/3 of the nucleus (hence the term " Ring Sideroblasts"). 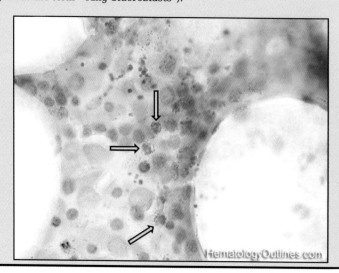

Rouleaux formation (rouleaux RBCs)	Stacking of RBCs (like a stack of coins) which is usually due to an increase in the relatively positively charged blood proteins, such as immunoglobulins and fibrinogen which ultimately lead to a decrease in the zeta potential between the RBCs and ultimately increase the chance of RBCs sticking to eachother. Rouleaux formation can be seen in multiple myeloma, and certain inflammatory conditions. 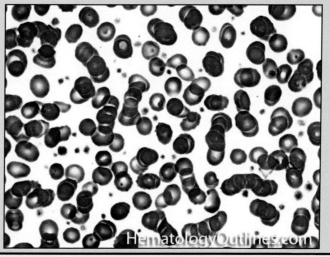
Russell bodies	Russell bodies are immunoglobin containing inclusions found in cytoplasm of plasma cells. They can be seen in multiple myeloma but they can also be seen in reactive non-neoplastic plasma cells. 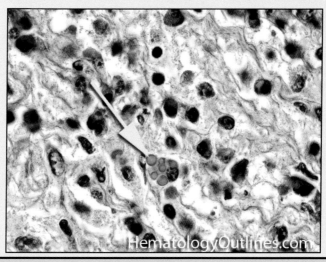
Russell Viper Venom Time	Also known as Dilute Russell Viper Venom Time (dRVVT), it is an in vitro qualitative test for lupus anticoagulant (LA) and usually follows an elevated PTT when LA is suspected. The test is derived from the venom of Russell viper, a power thrombotic agent in vitro. A mixing study is performed combining Russell's viper venom, patient's plasma, and phospholipids, which is required for coagulation. The presence of Lupus Anticoagulant would prevent clotting. A prolonged clotting time would be followed up with a confirmatory test where excess phospholipids are added to the mixing study, which should overcome LA and induce clotting. A ratio between clotting time without excess phospholipids and with excess phospholids is then calculated. An elevated ratio is considered positive and consistent with LA.

Schistocytes	These are irregularly shaped assymetrical fragmented RBCs that may have several morphologic forms (e.g. helmet cells, etc.). It is usually the result of mechanical disruption of the RBCs and many of which are generated by getting stuck to fibrin strands within the vessel wall (intravascular destruction) which may be secondary to a Microangiopathic hemolytic anemia such as HUS, TTP and DIC or a fibrin-independent destructive path such as being broken up by a mechanical heart valve. 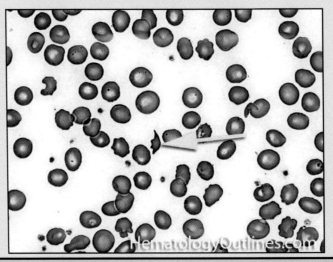
Segmented neutrophils	A segmented neutrophil is also referred to as a polymorphonuclear neutrophil (PMN). In a normal CBC, they are the most abundant white blood cells. They are also the first responders recruited to the site of injury such as inflammation which may be secondary to a bacterial infection, environmental exposure, and some cancers. 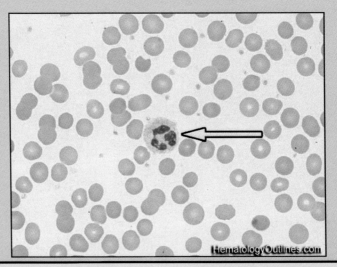
Sézary syndrome	Sézary syndrome is defined as a constellation of 1) erythroderma (with involvement by a cutaneous T-cell lymphoma which is usually comprised of CD4(+) T-cells), 2) circulating abnormal T-cells in the blood (Sézary cells) and 3) lymphadenopathy. On peripheral blood smear these Sézary cells are the abnormal lymphocytes with nuclear membrane irregularities and scant cytoplasm. When compared to the most common cutaneous T-cell lymphoma (mycoses fungoides), Sézary syndrome patients have a much worse prognosis.

Sickle cell	Abnormal RBCs seen in sickle cell anemia, with a rigid sickle shape and reduced flexibility. They have a banana shaped appearance. See sickle cell anemia. 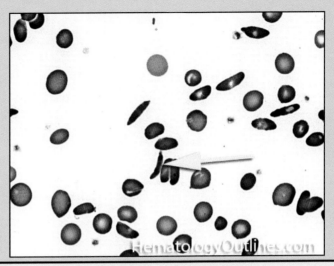
Sickle cell anemia	A hemoglobinopathy that is due to homozygosity from a point mutation in the beta-globin gene, where ultimately the glutamic acid (a hydrophilic residue) on position 6 of the beta globin chain is replaced with valine (a hydrophobic residue). The hydrophobic residues are not well suited for the surrounding hydrophilic environment inside the RBC and ultimately lead to aggregation of these abnormal hemoglobin molecules . These "polymerized" hemoglobin molecules cause abnormal RBCs with rigid and sickled shapes. Sickle cells lack the flexibility of normal RBCs and can be trapped within capillaries causing multiple complications (e.g. "sickle cell crisis" which includes vaso-occlusive crisis, hemolytic crisis, aplastic crisis, and sequestration crisis). Sickle cell patients commonly undergo autosplenetcomy during childhood due to infarction of the spleen with subsequent increased risk for developing infections due to encapsulated bacteria such as Streptococcus and H. influenzae, therefore requiring vaccinations. Various other clinical complications include stroke, avascular necrosis, osteomyelitis (Salmonella infection), chronic pain, pulmonary hypertension, chronic renal failure, and etc. 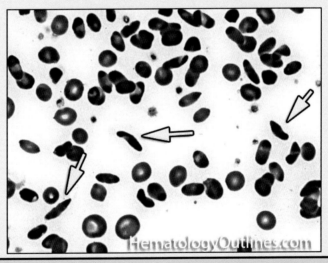
Sideroblastic anemia	A disease in which the bone marrow produces sideroblasts rather than normal RBC precursors. It can be caused by a genetic disorder or acquired such as in lead poisoning, zinc excess or sometimes seen with some myelodysplastic syndromes. In sideroblasic anemia, the body cannot properly utilize and incorporate iron into hemoglobin, therefore leading to an excess iron accumulation. The MCV is usually microcytic in sideroblastic anemia due to lead poisoning or congenital sideroblastic anemia while those associated with MDS can be macrocytic.
Sideroblasts	These are nucleated RBCs with a perinuclear deposition of iron granules. A type of these sideroblasts is called ring sideroblasts which can be seen in certain MDS such as Refractory Anemia with Ring Sideroblasts.

Small lymphocytic lymphoma	Also known as SLL, it is an indolent B-cell lymphoma and in simple terms chronic lymphocytic leukemia (CLL) involving tissue such as lymph nodes (hence the term lymphoma) . The characteristic immunophenotype is similar to CLL showing dim CD20 (+), CD19 (+), CD5 (+), CD23 (+), CD10 (-), and monotypic dim surface kappa or lambda light chain restricted neoplastic B-cells. 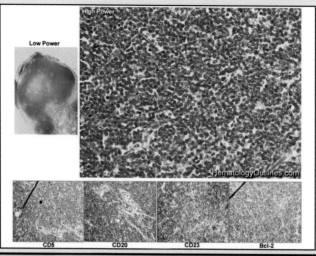
Smudge cells	Fragile lymphocytes that are broken down during blood smear preparation. Smudge cells are commonly seen in CLL. 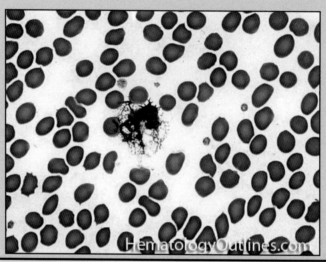
SPEP	Serum Protein Electrophoresis is a method that is used to separate and quantitate the different protein components of blood. One of these include the immunoglobulins, and when an M-spike (Monoclonal immunoglobulin band) is seen in this region on the gel, the amount of this potential clonal M-spike is quantitated by this method. Further charcaterization of this clone is done by IFE.
Spherocytes	Sphere shaped erythrocytes (RBCs) with reduced membrane and diameter which can be due to hereditary spherocytosis or autoimmune hemolytic anemia when increased numbers are noted in the peripheral blood. 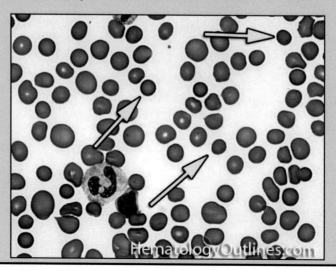

Splenic marginal zone lymphoma	A low-grade mature B-cell lymphoma that usually involves the spleen, peripheral blood and sometimes other organs such as the bone marrow. Characteristic features are splenomegaly (involving the white pulp of spleen as opposed to hairy cell leukemia which involves the splenic red pulp), moderate lymphocytosis with villous morphology (seen in the peripheral blood smear), and intrasinusoidal pattern of involvement of various organs, especially the bone marrow. Characteristic immunophenotype is similar to other marginal zone lymphomas (triple negative phenotype referring to being negative for CD5, CD10 and CD23). 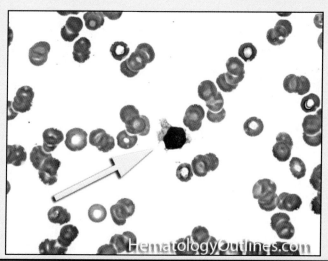
Splenomegaly	Splenomegaly is an enlargement of the spleen. Common causes of splenomegaly include infectious mononucleosis, end stage liver disease, certain hemoglobinopathies (e.g. HbSC disease), certain hematological malignancies (Many Myeloproliferitive Neoplasms, some lymphomas/leukemias such as splenic marginal zone lymphoma and hairy cell leukemia), infiltration by cancer, and certain metabolic diseases.
Spur cell RBC	Also known as acanthocyte, it is a RBC with irregular thorn-like projections. Looks like "Cowboy Boot Spurs". These RBCs may be associated with many conditions including but not limited to abetalipoproteinemia, liver disease, malnutrition, asplenia, and Mcleod phenotype blood group. 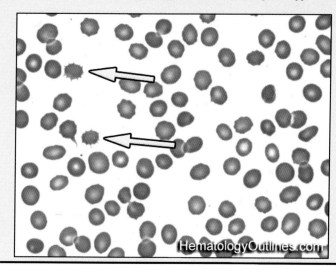

Stomatocytes	Stomatocytes are erythrocytes with a loosely folded, mouth-like pale area across the cell. They can be seen in hereditary stomatocytosis, liver disease, Rh null phenotypes, and Tangier's disease.
T-ALL	Also known as T-Lymphoblastic leukemia/lymphoma (or T-Acute lymphoblastic leukemia), it is an acute leukemia of lymphoid origin (specifically T-cell origin). Many involve the anterior mediastinum (thymus). Recall the mnemonic of 4 "Ts" for anterior mediastinal lesions: T for Terrible lymphomas (e.g. T-ALL, although Hodgkin lymphoma many times may involve anterior mediastinum and is not as aggressive as T-ALL), T for Thymoma, T for Thyroid remnant, and T for Teratoma (or other germ cell neoplasms).
T-cell	T-cells (also known as T-lymphocyte) are white blood cells involved in cell-mediated immunity along with other cells such as NK cells, etc. T-cell maturation (positive and negative selection) takes place within the Thymus (Remember T for T-cell and T for Thymus). Main subtypes of T-cells include, T-helper cells (CD4+) and cytotoxic T-cells (CD8+).
T-cell lymphomas	T-cell lymphomas are a group of Non-Hodgkin lymphomas (NHLs) that are the result of proliferating neoplastic T-lymphocytes (T-cells). They account for approximately 15% of the NHL group. Some of the more common types of T-cell lymphomas include Peripheral T-cell lymphoma NOS, Angioimmunoblastic T-cell lymphoma, Cutaneous T-cell lymphomas (most are Mycoises Fungoides), Anaplastic large cell lymphoma (ALCL), T-LGL leukemia and Adult T-cell lymphoma/leukemia (ATLL).

Target cells	Target cells are RBCs that resemble a bullseye; commonly seen in patients with thalassemia, certain hemoglobinopaties (e.g. Hb C disease), or even liver disease but can also be due to an artifact seen on certain peripheral blood smears secondary to slow drying of blood or excess EDTA.
Teardrop RBCs	Teardrop cells (dacrocytes) are RBCs that resemble a teardrop in the peripheral blood smear. They are often seen in people with an underlying myelofibrosis or other marrow space occupying disorders.
Thalassemia	A family of inherited blood disorders that is characterized by decreased production of either alpha or beta-globin chains of the hemoglobin molecule. The two major types of thalassemias are alpha thalassemia (decreased alpha chain production) and beta thalassemia (decreased beta chain production). The decreased hemoglobin production results in microcytic anemia.
Thrombopoietin	A protein (hormone) produced by the liver and kidney that stimulates production and differentiation of megakaryocytes and ultimately stimulates the production of more platelets. Note: "Thrombo" refers to platelets and "-poietin" refers to its ability to stimulate production.
Thrombotic Thrombocytopenic Purpura	Also known as TTP, it is a microangiopathic hemolytic anemia that is typically due to deficiency of ADAMTS-13 (a metalloprotease responsible for cleavage of large multimers of vW factor). Similar to HUS remember the mnemonic "Brain FART" (complements of Dr. M. Baughn) which is "Brain" for the neurologic problems (more commonly associated with TTP than HUS), F for Fever, A for Anemia, R for Renal failure (more commonly associated with HUS than TTP), and T for the Thrombocytopenia.
Thymocyte	An immature T-cell in the thymus. The sequential thymocyte stages can be defined by their location in the thymus (e.g. cortical thymocyte, medullary thymocyte). The stages can also be divided immunophenotypically into CD4/CD8 double negative, CD4/CD8 double positive, and single positive CD4 or CD8. T-cell receptor (TCR) genes rearrangement takes place in the thymus in these thymocytes as they mature into functional CD4+ or CD8+ T-cells.
Tissue Factor	Also known as platelet tissue factor and Factor III. A cell surface protein present on subendothelial cells, platelets, and leukocytes. As a part of extrinsic coagulation pathway, TF contains a receptor which binds Factor VIIa which then converts Factor X to Xa, activating the common coagulation pathway.

Vitamin K	Fat-soluble vitamin required in coagulation and metabolic pathways. The Vitamin K dependent Coagulation factors are II, VII, IX, X, protein C and protein S.
von Willebrand Disease	A hereditary or acquired coagulation disorder resulting from either a qualitative change of vWF (usually a mutation giving rise to an abnormal vWF) or quantitative deficiency of vWF. There are three types of hereditary vWF deficiencies: Type 1, Type 2, and Type 3. Type 1 is the most common form and is a quantitative defect where vWF are decreased. Most patients are asymptomatic; however, symtoms such as prolonged bleeding post-surgery, menorrhagia, or easy bruising can occur. Type 2 is subdivided into 2A, 2B, 2M, and 2N, and it is a qualitative defect of vWF. Type 2B is unique in that the mutation leads to an increased binding of platelets to vWF and increased clearance thus producing a mild thrombocytopenia. Type 2M and 2N are rare. Type 3 is the most severe form and has no detectable levels of vWF.
von Willebrand Factor	Also known as vWF, it is a multimeric protein produced in the endothelium and subendothelial tissues, and also in the alpha granules within platelets. vWF is bound to Factor VIII while inactive and released by the influence of thrombin and binds to subendothelial collagen during vessel trauma and damage. vWF then binds to platelets via the GPIb receptor. Additional platelets bind via vWF and the process repeats. The breakdown of vWF multimers is by ADAMTS13, a metalloproteinase.
vWF	Also known as Von Willebrand Factor, it is a multimeric protein produced in the endothelium and subendothelial tissues, and also in the alpha granules within platelets. vWF is bound to Factor VIII while inactive and released by the influence of thrombin and binds to subendothelial collagen during vessel trauma and damage. vWF then binds to platelets via the GPIb receptor. Additional platelets bind via vWF and the process repeats. The breakdown of vWF multimers is by ADAMTS13, a metalloproteinase.
Waldenstrom's macroglobulinemia	Waldenstrom's macroglobulinemia (WM) is a clinical disease usually caused by an increase in abnormal B-lymphocytes which produce increased amounts of monoclonal immunoglobulins (typically IgM). Very high levels of IgM in the blood may cause hyperviscosity , which could explain the symptoms associated with this disease (blurred vision, headache, and dizziness). The lymphoma that is most commonly associated with WM is lymphoplasmacytic lymphoma (a low grade B-cell lymphoma).
WBC	White blood cells are the nucleated cells noted in the peripheral blood as part of a CBC and include neutrophils, lymphocytes, monocytes, eosinophils, and basophils (in order of prevalence).
White Blood Cells	Also known as WBC, these are the nucleated cells noted in the peripheral blood as part of a CBC and include neutrophils, lymphocytes, monocytes, eosinophils, and basophils (in order of prevalence).
Zeta potential	The electrical potential difference between red blood cells created by the surface negative charges on the red blood cells and the surrounding cations in the blood. This repulsive force prevents the RBCs from sticking together under normal conditions. Conditions that decrease this repulsion are typically relatively positively charged molecules which increases the chance of RBC agglutination (e.g. increased Ig levels as in plasma cell myeloma or changing the ionic strength when adding Low Ionic Strength Solution (LISS) in certain blood bank tests, etc.)

Notes:

Index:

References:

Arber DA, Orazi A, Hasserjian R, Thiele J, Borowitz MJ, Le Beau MM, Bloomfield CD, Cazzola M, Vardiman JW. The 2016 revision to the World Health Organization classification of myeloid neoplasms and acute leukemia. Blood. 2016 May 19;127(20):2391-405.

Campo E, Swerdlow SH, Harris NL, Pileri S, Stein H, Jaffe ES. The 2008 WHO classification of lymphoid neoplasms and beyond: evolving concepts and practical applications. Blood. 2011 May 12;117(19):5019-32.

Gabrilove J. Overview: erythropoiesis, anemia, and the impact of erythropoietin. Semin Hematol. 2000 Oct;37(4 Suppl 6):1-3.

Gorczyca W. Flow cytometry immunophenotypic characteristics of monocytic population in acute monocytic leukemia (AML-M5), acute myelomonocytic leukemia (AML-M4), and chronic myelomonocytic leukemia (CMML). Methods Cell Biol. 2004;75:665-77.

Gorczyca W, Sun ZY, Cronin W, Li X, Mau S, Tugulea S. Immunophenotypic pattern of myeloid populations by flow cytometry analysis. Methods Cell Biol. 2011;103:221-66.

Swerdlow SH, Campo E, Harris NL, Jaffe ES, Pileri S, Stein H, Thiele J, Vardiman JW. WHO Classification of Tumours of Haematopoietic and Lymphoid Tissues. 4th edition, IARC: Lyon, 2008.

Swerdlow SH, Campo E, Pileri SA, Harris NL, Stein H, Siebert R, Advani R, Ghielmini M, Salles GA, Zelenetz AD, Jaffe ES. The 2016 revision of the World Health Organization classification of lymphoid neoplasms. Blood. 2016 May 19;127(20):2375-90.